Praise for *Staying Clean and Sober*

"Thank you, Millers, for putting in one convenient book everything we tell the clients at Sacramento County Drug Court, and more! You've created not only a sourcebook for people tired of 'white-knuckling' their way through recovery, but also for those of us providing treatment who know that brain repair is the essential first step to release anyone from any addiction."
—Carolyn Reuben, LAc, author of *Cleansing the Body, Mind, and Spirit*, and President, Community Addiction Recovery Association

"A courageous step forward from two pioneers in the substance abuse field who have worked long and hard to present this new technology with a great voice. This important work in the integration of alternative treatment modalities for chemical dependency is long overdue."
—Stan Stokes, Executive Director of Bridging the Gaps

"The Millers are exceptional communicators and educators in the addiction field. This book offers groundbreaking, life-saving information for anyone involved in recovery."
—Dr. James Braly, author of *Dr. Braly's Food Allergy and Nutrition Revolution*

"Merlene and David are far ahead of their time. They are among the first to finally change the way we treat addiction in this country."
—Tamea Sisco, DD, CAd

Other Books by Merlene Miller and David Miller

Reversing the Regression Spiral
Merlene Miller and David Miller

Staying Sober: A Guide for Relapse Prevention
Terence T. Gorski and Merlene Miller

*Learning to Live Again: A Guide for Recovery
from Chemical Dependency*
Merlene Miller, Terence Gorski, and David Miller

*Overload: Attention Deficit Disorder and
the Addictive Brain*
David Miller and Kenneth Blum

Reversing the Weight Gain Spiral
Merlene Miller and David Miller

How to Quit
Patrick Holford, David Miller, and James Braly

Counseling for Relapse Prevention
Terence Gorski and Merlene Miller

Staying Clean and Sober

Staying Clean and Sober

Complementary and Natural Strategies for Healing the Addicted Brain

Third Edition

MERLENE MILLER, MA AND DAVID MILLER, PHD

In Collaboration with Kenneth Blum, PhD

Note: The information in this book is for educational purposes only and is not recommended as a means of diagnosing or treating an illness. All matters concerning physical and mental health should be supervised by a health practitioner knowledgeable in treating that particular condition. Neither the publisher nor the authors directly or indirectly dispense medical advice, nor do they prescribe any remedies or assume any responsibility for those who choose to treat themselves.

For more information on some of the therapies mentioned in this book or copies of this book call: **800-614-7714**

ISBN-13: 9781541323223
ISBN-10: 154132322X

In loving memory of Sue Sloan

Contents

Acknowledgments

We have had help in writing this book. And the message we share reflects the words and works of the dedicated people we consider part of our team. First of all, we want to thank Kenneth Blum for his pioneering work in bringing much of the information in this book to light. And specifically we thank him for his contributions to this book, especially in chapters two and five. We also want to thank the other people who have shared our vision of more effective treatment. We appreciate the work of Stan Stokes, Jim Braly, Julia Ross, Doug Sloan, Jan Sloan, Charles Gant, Carol Cummings, Dee Ogle, Matt and Debra Manka, Pat Smith, Diana and Richard Guthrie, Bill Hitt, Anne Brady, Irene Dowler, Terry Gorski, Lisa Havens, Marilyn Shank, Terri Rathbun, Anne Barcus, and Carolyn Reuben. The voices of these people are in this book and their work has led the way and guided us in our search for better treatment. Thanks to those who assisted in manuscript preparation: Teah Sloan, Paul Kennard, Stephanie von Hirschberg, and Jane Heywood. We are grateful to special friends who have supported us through our journey. Our wonderful family is always supportive and assists us in any way they can. Thanks to our sons, our daughter-in-law, and our grandchildren.

One

OUR STORY: THE SEARCH FOR BETTER TREATMENT

When I met David Miller, he was an active alcoholic. I didn't recognize it because, as he has often said, I knew so little about alcoholism that I thought withdrawal was talking with a southern accent. I thought he drank too much, but as I wasn't planning to marry him, I figured it was his business. But both those factors changed. What had been a close friendship developed into a deep love, and a life crisis caused him to make the decision to quit drinking. As far as I was concerned, the drinking problem was over and we were in love, so we got married.

His period of abstinence didn't last very long. And living with his drinking instead of observing it as an outsider was more of a problem than I knew how to deal with. I had four children from a previous marriage, and ultimately I felt I had to ask him to choose between us and his drinking. He chose us and began attending Alcoholics Anonymous. But his decision to stop drinking was just the beginning of our struggles. I thought that if he weren't drinking everything would be fine. I didn't realize that there are symptoms of addiction that emerge with abstinence that can make life nearly as uncomfortable as the drinking. (Most authorities now think these symptoms precede and contribute to addiction in the first place.)

Without alcohol David was moody, stress sensitive, and irritable. He was highly sensitive to noise (and all of my children are hearing impaired, resulting in a noisier than usual environment); and he sometimes found family life almost unbearable. He often withdrew from the rest of us, leaving me feeling depressed and rejected. Sometimes I thought it had been easier to live with him when he was drinking.

Despite this, I respected his effort to maintain sobriety even when I could see it was extremely difficult for him. I tried to be supportive, and he tried to give as much to the marriage as he was able. But sometimes the internal turmoil became so unbearable that he drank. For three years, he struggled to maintain sobriety (and periodically slipped) before he was able to maintain ongoing abstinence. He now has forty years of continuous recovery.

David's years of sobriety are due somewhat to what we learned together about managing what we later called chronic abstinence symptoms of addiction. In all the meetings we attended, all the counseling we received, and all the reading we did, no one told us it would be so difficult. No one told us that these symptoms are frequently part of recovery. And no one told us what to do about them because, quite frankly, no one really knew.

We learned by trial and error to cope with David's symptoms. For instance, we noticed that the symptoms were worse on Saturdays. Why? As we looked at what was different we found a number of culprits. He slept later on Saturdays, thus ate later. In fact, he would often get up and go to his AA sponsor's house without eating. There he would drink coffee, eat donuts, and smoke cigarettes. And when he came home, he would find me vacuuming, the kids playing music, the phone ringing, and general chaos reigning. His only way of coping was to leave, which I resented. So when he did come back, even if things had settled down, I was usually not in a loving, supportive mood.

Eventually, because our desire to make our marriage better was so strong, we began to search for answers to the problems linked to David's fight with abstinence. Some of the steps we took were very simple. I began taking a glass of orange juice to him before he got out of bed to raise his blood sugar (and, though I didn't realize it at the time, to temporarily alter his brain chemistry). He started eating breakfast before he went to see his sponsor and refrained from the donuts and limited the coffee. Almost immediately, he was amazed at how different he felt. When he came home he was in a better mood, and I tried to reduce the typical noise and clamor. David made more of an effort to stick around and contribute to the Saturday needs of the family. But if things did become too stressful I tried to understand his need to get away for a time.

Gradually, David and I found other ways to help him maintain a more comfortable sobriety. We found ways to reduce noise levels in the home. We discovered that you can't just work at recovery. You have to play, too. We found that there must be creative and enjoyable activities to replace the void left by the absence of alcohol. What we were doing, but didn't realize at the time, was finding ways to alter the chemicals in the brain that help us feel good.

Because of our efforts, we were not only able to hold our marriage together, but we also built a stronger relationship by working together to figure out how to live in sobriety. The point of this story is that long-term, lasting sobriety is difficult. It is not just a matter of will-power and self-discipline. It is not just a choice to stop using and go on with your life. What we came to understand was that addiction is a physiologically and biochemically linked condition and that there are physiological and biochemical symptoms that can't be ignored. We realized that when recovering addicts relapse it is usually not because they don't want to stay sober. *It's because they don't know how.*

What we learned by our own trial and error, and a lot of heartache, we wanted to share with other people in recovery. We determined to help others find alternatives to relapse and to the pain that often accompanies abstinence. To do that, we began looking for better and better ways to smooth out the road to recovery.

After a few years of ongoing recovery, David went back to school and became an addiction counselor. He was fortunate to work with Terry Gorski, who was also interested in relapse prevention. Terry was looking at what he called post-acute withdrawal, a group of symptoms he had found often accompanied abstinence. It was a relief to have a name for the symptoms David experienced and to realize that he was not alone. These symptoms are common in sobriety.

Together, Terry, David, and I wrote a book called *Learning to Live Again: A Guide to Recovery from Alcoholism* (later revised and called *Learning to Live Again: A Guide to Recovery from Chemical Dependency*). In this book we were able to share what we had learned about the road to recovery and how to make it smoother. And it was exciting to realize that other people could benefit from what we had learned the hard way.

Later, Terry and I wrote a book called *Staying Sober: A Guide to Relapse Prevention.* This book has been used widely in the addiction field since 1986. The reason for its wide acceptance is that people who read the book began learning for the first time about symptoms that make recovery difficult. They realize that they are not crazy or hopeless if they have these symptoms or if they relapse. What a relief.

In *Staying Sober* we say that post-acute withdrawal symptoms are due to damage to the nervous system from drug use and will go away as the brain and body heal. But what began to trouble David after a time was that for many people the symptoms never go away. They had never gone away for him. He had just learned how to cope with them. But after more than ten years of sobriety, these effects could still make him very uncomfortable.

Eventually David and I had our own treatment program, and clients told us they still suffered from symptoms after many years of sobriety. Because we specialized in relapse prevention, most of the people we saw struggled with the symptoms and with periodic relapse. We realized that for some people recovery is not a road to travel but a mountain to climb. We developed our own strategy of relapse prevention and applied it to a variety of conditions, including food addiction. We wrote a book, *Reversing the Weight Gain Spiral*, about preventing relapse by compulsive overeaters.

As we taught clients about post-acute withdrawal symptoms, many of them told us that they had experienced the symptoms *before* they started drinking or using drugs (or overeating). They had the symptoms as long as they could remember. And they told us that these symptoms were the reason they started drinking or using drugs in the first place as self-medication for their discomfort.

David became convinced that what we were calling post- acute withdrawal, in many cases, was not really withdrawal but the return of symptoms that had been relieved by using addictive substances. He was especially sure of this in relation to the symptoms of heightened sensitivity to noise and lights and even touch. He began to learn more about this symptom, often called stimulus augmentation, or sometimes hyper-augmentation or hypersensitivity. His interest was further heightened because he had been plagued with this condition since he was a child.

David found that most chronic relapsers experienced stimulus augmentation. He discovered that people with attention deficit hyperactivity disorder (ADHD) frequently have this symptom and that people with ADHD often have alcohol and drug problems. He was ultimately diagnosed with attention deficit disorder himself and later, with Dr. Kenneth Blum, wrote the book *Overload: Attention Deficit Disorder and the Addictive Brain*. Through further research, David also discovered that many people in recovery from addiction have undiagnosed ADHD. As he continued his study, he found that there are other related disorders that predispose people to addiction, among them Tourette's syndrome, obsessive-compulsive disorder, depression, and conduct disorder. All these conditions are neurological and biochemical, meaning they are related to chemical imbalances in the brain. The more David and I analyzed the research related to addiction, the more aware we became of the gap between what is known about addiction and what is being done about it. As scientific research has taught us more and more about the nature of addiction, treatment has not changed—or has changed very little—to utilize this information.

If addiction is related to brain chemistry, then it seemed to us that to effectively treat addiction we had to find more effective and natural ways to alter the brain's chemistry. David and I began investigating alternative therapies that could be used to restore healthy brain chemistry, thereby aiding addicts in their recovery: nutrition, auricular therapy, acupuncture, and brain-wave biofeedback (neurofeedback) are but a few.

David started taking an amino acid supplement formulated by Dr. Kenneth Blum. The results were amazing—he experienced significant relief from his symptoms. This made perfect sense because brain chemicals are produced, in large part, from amino acids and vitamins, and addiction and ADHD are related to brain chemistry.

Because of the remarkable changes resulting from taking the amino acid formulation, David began recommending the amino acid supplement to addiction clients, most of whom also got positive results. The right combination of amino acids and vitamins delivered to the brain of the addict can restore the balance of neurotransmitters, bringing a sense of well-being and relief from craving.

While searching for more effective treatments, we found that other neurological treatments are currently being used successfully to help people overcome the craving for alcohol or drugs. Hundreds of drug courts throughout the United States have found that auriculotherapy or ear acupuncture, is more effective than traditional methods alone. Brain-wave biofeedback (neurofeedback) has been found to be effective in changing brain-wave patterns so individuals have the power to choose to increase brain waves that help them relax or concentrate better. Many people find therapeutic massage to be relaxing, soothing, and good for the body.

Somewhere in our journey to find better treatment for the physical symptoms of addiction, we began to lose sight of the importance of the psychological and spiritual needs of the recovering person. We began to observe that when people relied on amino acid therapy, acupuncture or neurofeedback alone they were more likely to relapse. We realized that treating the brain alone without addressing emotional and spiritual needs was as incomplete as treatment that does not provide healing for the brain.

As more scientific information about the biochemical nature of addiction has become available in recent years, we have seen a growing tendency to treat it with prescription medications. While medications do address the physiology of addiction, we see this as a step in the wrong direction. In most cases, medications do not treat the underlying problem. Medications often have side effects that become problems themselves or cause the person to stop taking them. Medications can become new addictions. Perhaps most important, certain medications pose a danger if people relapse and drink or use while taking them. The resulting reaction between the drug(s) and the addictive substance can be very harmful, even fatal. For these reasons, we do not present prescription medication as a recommended strategy for healing the addicted brain. Medications should only be used as a last resort, and then with a great deal of caution.

This book is the culmination of what we have learned so far about complete and lasting addiction recovery. We have searched for explanations as to why addiction recovery is so difficult as well as for treatments that could make recovery easier. This is what we have come to believe as a result of our journey: Addiction is primarily a disease of the brain, and the biochemical imbalances associated with it create chronic abstinence symptoms that often lead to relapse. For many people, unless healthy brain chemistry is restored, staying sober and drug-free means living with emotional pain—anxiety, confusion, and depression. Treatment that addresses only the psychological, social, and spiritual issues related to addiction is effective less than 20 percent of the time. Complete treatment for addiction requires combining treatment for the brain with counseling and education to support lifestyle change. Alternative therapies for healing the brain are being used with great success—in particular, nutritional and amino acid therapy with a recovery rate of 70 to 75 percent—but, unfortunately, few people know about them. Healing of the brain must be supported by healing of the spirit. Self-care and relapse prevention are essential for comfortable ongoing sobriety.

We are witnessing the birth of what we have been searching for. We are entering a new era of treatment. The work being done now is pioneer work, and, for us, the search for more effective treatment goes on.

Perhaps you suffer from alcoholism or drug addiction and have found no effective treatment. Perhaps you are a parent, husband, wife, son, daughter, or friend of an addict and are living a life of quiet desperation, believing your loved one is hopelessly addicted and can never return to healthful living. Perhaps you are an addiction professional (doing everything you know to do to give life back to people who are addicted) facing, day after day, the reality that the large majority of your addicted clients are relapsing because the treatment you offer has not provided relief from the discomfort that often accompanies abstinence. We hope the message of this book will open the door to new options and new hope for you.

By Merlene Miller

Two

This Is Your Brain on Drugs: This Is Your Life on Drugs

According to the American Society of Addiction Medicine (ASAM), addiction is a disorder of the brain.[1] It results from and leads to low levels of dopamine, a chemical in the brain that plays a significant role in feelings of motivation, cognition, pleasure, and well-being. As we explain this, you may find it hard to digest if you are unfamiliar with some of the scientific terms. But try to stay with us. We want you to know that what we are telling you is based on scientific research and is not just someone's idea or theory. To show you this, we need to tell you about the research behind what we know about the brain and addiction. The person most responsible for this research is Dr. Kenneth Blum. Almost half a century of addiction research extends from double-blind placebo-controlled studies to neuro-imaging.

It is important for you to know how and why people become addicted and what can be done about it.[2] No one intends to become addicted. No child says, "I'm going to be an alcoholic when I grow up." No adolescent who experiments with drugs thinks, "I want to become a junkie." No one, when taking the first puff, drink, sniff, or injection, plans on getting addicted to cigarettes, alcohol, marijuana, glue, speed, cocaine, prescription medications, bath salts, or heroin.

Yet for a great number of people, that first deceptive drink or hit leads to addictive behaviors and physical dependence. In fact, when one's initial response to the first drink or hit is very memorable, it indicates the possibility of a genetic marker for being in high risk for all addictive behaviors. It is impossible for anyone who has never been addicted to comprehend the power of addiction. It seems logical and reasonable to stop doing something so harmful to yourself and others, especially those you care about most.

But addicts think about drug use, not with the part of their brain that is reasonable and logical, but with the part that is concerned with survival: the limbic system, the part that tells us to eat, drink, flee, or fight. The limbic system is concerned with keeping us alive. It monitors the body's need for survival, and when it senses that our survival is dependent on a certain behavior, it creates a compulsion so strong that it becomes extremely difficult to resist taking that action. Without that compulsion, we might forget to eat or reproduce. The limbic system tells addicts that they must have the addictive substance or they will die (and in some cases, that is true). The limbic system controls the thinking of the addicted person even after the pleasure of drinking or taking drugs has been replaced by severe pain.

There is another part of the brain called the pre-frontal lobe that is known to control cognition, and, even more, importantly "decision-making."[3] If your brain is not able to perform this function appropriately, your judgment will be poor and you will be set up to make wrong decisions.

It is now known that this part of the brain does not fully develop until in the mid 20's. This means that adolescents, because of poor judgment coupled with peer pressure, are at higher risk to experiment with drugs. When there is also an inherited genetic risk for addiction, it can lead to unstoppable drug-abuse. The limbic site is where craving resides and the pre-frontal site is where judgment occurs.[4]

Patty, a cocaine addict, struggling unsuccessfully to overcome her addiction, describes it this way: It seems like I have two brains. There is the brain that tells me that if I use cocaine, I am going to be miserable; it's not fun anymore; it's not worth it; afterward I will feel guilt and remorse and I am deeper in debt. The other brain says that I really need this; I have to have it; something worse than death will happen to me if I don't have it; I deserve it, and, this time, I might get back the old feeling that I need so badly. This argument goes on until the brain, in favor of using cocaine, convinces the other one that I probably will end up doing it anyway, so I may as well go ahead and do it early so I won't be up all night and unable to work the next day. For some reason, this makes sense to my other brain and I go get some coke.

But how does a person get to the point where the survival part of the brain overrules the reasoning part? And why does it happen to some people who drink alcohol, smoke marijuana, or try cocaine and not to others who do the same thing?

James and Richard are brothers we have known since they were young. As teenagers, they used drugs together. They used the same drugs in the same quantities. But as they reached college age, James realized that his drug use was interfering with what he wanted out of life. He quit using illegal drugs though he continued to drink infrequently and always in moderation. By the same age, Richard realized that what he wanted out of life *was* drugs.

James enrolled in college, established a career, had a family, and became a respected, politically active member of his community. Richard also enrolled in college—many times in fact—but he never completed a semester before some drug-related incident interfered and caused him to drop out. He married a couple of times, but when his wives asked him to choose between them and drugs, he chose drugs. He eventually went to prison and served an eighteen-month sentence for possession of cocaine.

While their upbringing was similar, what was different between these brothers? Why did they take such different paths despite the outward similarities in their early drug use? To answer this, we need to examine what normally happens in the brain, and what differs in some people that causes them to be more susceptible to using and becoming addicted to mood-altering substances.

The Brain Reward Cascade (The Happy Brain)

We all want to feel good. We seek physical and emotional comfort. When our needs are met, our brain *rewards* us. It's as simple as that. Adequate food, water, and sleep act as a stimulus that activates a chemical reaction in the brain that rewards us with a feeling of satisfaction. A word of praise for a job well done or a hug from a loved one sets off a brain chemical interaction that feels good. What produces these rewards is different for different people. Chocolate may produce more reward for one person while potato chips may produce more reward for someone else. Reading a novel may be rewarding for someone, while, skiing may be rewarding for another. We all differ in what gives us satisfaction and in the depth of satisfaction we experience, and this could be due to our genes. [5]

Different parts of the brain communicate to keep us alive and happy. We have already talked about the survival and decision-making part of the brain. The "reward" and memory parts of the brain also play important roles in addiction. When you are hungry, the reward site of the brain tells the survival part to find something to satisfy the hunger. When you eat food that tastes good and fills your stomach, dopamine is released into the reward site and gives you a jolt of pleasure. That's your reward for eating.

When you eat, the memory of the reward is stored in another part of the brain. The brain remembers that certain behaviors result in good feelings and other behaviors result in bad feelings. It remembers that when you were hungry, you felt bad and when you had adequate food you felt satisfied. That memory motivates you to eat again.

Neurotransmitters are the chemical messengers that mediate mood, emotion, thought, behavior, motivation, and memories. Neurotransmitters work together to create feelings of pleasure to reward us for certain behaviors that help keep us alive and comfortable. The actions we take in response to the drives to eat, drink, have sex or seek pleasurable activities lead to the release of the neurotransmitter dopamine into the area of the brain called the nucleus accumbens (often referred to as the reward area). By giving us a reward, the brain works to ensure that we will repeat behaviors necessary for us to survive and transfer our DNA from one generation to the next. It rewards us for normal behaviors that we need to repeat to stay alive, be healthy, reproduce, and feel pleasure.[6]

Neurotransmitters act as stimulators and inhibitors in our brains that act upon one another in a way that typically creates an adequate supply of dopamine. Kenneth Blum refers to this chemical interaction as the "brain reward cascade." When this process works as nature intends, this chemical cascade results in feelings of pleasure and well being. Here is how it works.

This figure represents neurons, neurotransmitters, neurotransmitter receptors and the areas of the reward system of the brain where the complex interactions that result in the release of dopamine occur.

Manufactured and stored within brain cells (neurons), neurotransmitters carry messages from one neuron to another. When a neuron receives a stimulus (from something we see, hear, feel, taste, smell, think, imagine, or perceive), it sends a chemical message across a synapse (the space between neurons) to the next neuron, which sends the message on to the next. Reaching out like the branches of a tree, each neuron connects with thousands of others, all of which are sending and receiving chemical messages from one to another.

Once released, neurotransmitters seek out and attach to adjacent neurons that have receptors with a complementary shape. Neurotransmitters fit into these receptors the way a key fits into a lock, and receptors will accept only those neurotransmitters with a corresponding shape. Both neurotransmitters and receptors play a crucial role in our ability to feel pleasure. An adequate supply of dopamine and a sufficient number of receptors are necessary for a happy brain. To understand the nature of addiction, it is important to know that receptors will also accept ingested mood-altering chemicals that mimic natural brain chemicals.

Neurotransmitters are manufactured in the brain's neurons from amino acids (e.g. L-tryptophane, L-Tyrosine, DL-phenylalanine, L-Glutamine, etc.) There are at least five brain chemicals that play a significant role in who becomes addicted: *dopamine*, the primary neurotransmitter of reward; serotonin; opioid peptides (endorphins, enkephalins, and dynorphins) that we will refer to collectively as endorphins; and gamma-aminobutyric acid (GABA). These brain chemicals interact in a cascade that works like this.

Serotonin helps you relax *and stimulates the production of endorphins*

Endorphins relieve physical and emotional pain and *regulate the production of GABA.*

GABA reduces anxiety and *inhibits the production of dopamine.* (CAUTION: Excess GABA results in a pleasure deficit by inhibiting dopamine production.)

Dopamine released into the reward site of the brain is the final outcome of the reward cascade. A sufficient supply of dopamine gives us the reward we are seeking: feelings of pleasure and well-being. It increases alertness and energy.

Dopamine is the primary neurotransmitter of reward. It is the net release of dopamine that translates into a sense of well-being. When the reward system of the brain is working properly, it rewards us with a feeling of well-being, pleasure, and satiation from normal activities by releasing dopamine in the reward center of the brain. Endorphins, serotonin, and GABA work together to allow the optimal amount of dopamine to reward us with feelings of satisfaction and well-being. The number one goal in treating addiction is giving the brain the optimal amount of dopamine: "dopamine homeostasis."

This illustrates the interaction of neurotransmitters within the reward pathway of the brain. A homeostatic balance is maintained in the happy brain and adequate dopamine is released.

Reward Deficiency Syndrome

But what happens if and when this reward system does not work properly? Nora D. Volkow, the director of the National Institute on Drug Abuse (NIDA), has suggested that "all roads lead to dopamine." If this is the case, a "Happy Brain" requires just enough dopamine to feel good, and when there is low dopamine function, one may have an "Unhappy Brain." Kenneth Blum has coined the term *reward deficiency syndrome*[7] to describe a condition in which the reward system of the brain is not working properly and results in a lack of reward for normal, healthy activities. The body seeks a neurochemical balance, and when there is an imbalance leading to low dopamine, the brain sends out a powerful message to correct the imbalance. Lack of dopamine homeostasis can result in a reward deficiency that can manifest itself as restlessness, anxiety, emptiness, lack of satisfaction, and vague or specific cravings. These feelings are the brain's message to us to take action to correct the imbalance. People with reward deficiency may feel as if they are constantly in need of something to fill the emptiness, reduce the anxiety, elevate the mood, quiet the restlessness, or satisfy the cravings.

There are numerous causes of reward deficiency. Many people are born with one or more genetic impairments or variants that interfere with normal brain chemical interactions and balance. Numerous genes have been identified that are associated with conditions that manifest themselves as symptoms of reward deficiency. Among the genetic conditions, associated with reward deficiency, are ADHD, Tourette's syndrome, and obsessive-compulsive disorder. And this is a key point: Many people *born with a genetic reward deficiency are also genetically predisposed to addiction.*[8]

Andrea's father was alcoholic. Although she was not aware of it at the time, she realizes now that he also had ADHD. She was diagnosed with ADHD as an adult recovering alcoholic. In remembering her childhood, she recalls that she was always restless and anxious, had difficulty concentrating, was easily stressed, and was distracted by noise and competing sounds. She remembers that she never felt comfortable, at ease, or satisfied and believed there was something seriously wrong with her, but she had no idea what it was. She just knew from an early age that she was different. It wasn't until she discovered alcohol in her early teens and began using it to change her brain chemistry that she began to fit in and feel comfortable and satisfied.

After dopamine is released from the nerve cell, it interacts with a dopamine receptor (where it fits like a key in a lock). If too little dopamine is released or if there is a reduced number of dopamine receptors, the result is low dopamine function. It is important to remember that reduced dopamine function can be a result of too few receptors as well as low dopamine release. This suggests that our goal of creating dopamine homeostasis is not only to release dopamine but also to fix any deviation from normal in the number of dopamine receptors.

Many genes associated with addiction have been identified. The risk of addiction is very high among those who are genetically predisposed to having an abnormal form or variant of a gene called the dopamine D2 receptor gene (DRD2) which normally lays down dopamine receptors. Carriers of one form of the gene, called A1, have 30-40% fewer dopamine D2 receptors than those who carry the A2 form. What is remarkable is that Kenneth Blum and Ernest P. Noble, who first discovered the association between the A1 form and severe alcoholism, have also reported that in the United States alone over 100 million people carry the low dopamine receptor form (A1) leading to reward deficiency syndrome (RDS).[9]

In addition to the A1 form of the DRD2 gene, other gene variants can affect the net release of dopamine. For example, a gene known as the COMT gene is responsible for the breakdown of dopamine in the synapse. If an individual carries one form of this gene, the dopamine in the synapse is broken down four times faster than those that have other forms. This results in low dopamine and the subsequent lack of reward, providing the motivation to self-medicate with a mood-altering substance.

Certainly reward deficiency from non-genetic causes can also put a person at high risk for addiction. The reward cascade can be altered by environmental conditions as well as many gene variations. People may be at higher risk for addiction because of genetic factors (nature) or environmental factors (nurture) or a *combination of both*. Research suggests that genes and environment contribute equally to the risk for addiction. *Behavior equals our DNA plus our environment.*

While we have noted the role of environment on behavior, scientific exploration over the past decade has led to a better understanding of how the environment interacts with our DNA to cause addiction. We call this interaction *epigenetics*. More is now known about how the environment can, in fact, alter the expression of our genes.[10]

The leading figure in unraveling the mysteries of environmentally-induced genetic expression called *epigenetics* is Eric Nestler from Mount Sinai Medical School in NYC. The mechanism is quite complicated and involves chemical reactions that occur when there are positive and/or negative environmental stimuli. This effect can actually be passed from one generation to at least two subsequent generations. For example, poor parenting including child abuse may cause epigenetic effects leading to poor parenting and abuse in the next generation, This effect is due to shutting off expression of feel-good genes. In contrast, loving support from parents to their offspring can lead to an enhancement of gene expression. Even the risks associated with the A1 form of the DRD2 gene can be decreased with supportive parenting. So the lesson here according to Nester is that: Parents should love their children.

Non-genetic conditions can affect reward deficiency, with or without a genetic predisposition, these include:

Prenatal conditions such as alcohol use or drug use by the mother, malnutrition, exposure to toxins, or injury during pregnancy can result in a lifetime of impaired brain chemistry. In the late 70's Kenneth

Blum found that rodent prenatal exposure to the psychoactive ingredient in cannabis tetrahydrocannabinol (THC) induced a higher sensitivity to the effects of the stress-producing norepinephrine in the next generation of rats.

More recently animal work from Yasmin Hurd and associates at Mount Sinai Medical School has shown that parental exposure to THC is associated with changes in the expression of specific receptor genes in the reward center of the brain such that prenatal exposure leads to compulsive heroin seeking.[11]

Malnutrition over an extended period of time (caused by very-low-calorie dieting, the unavailability of food, food allergy/sensitivity, or a nutritionally inadequate diet) can impair the proper production and interaction of brain chemicals. Neurotransmitters are produced from amino acids, vitamins, and minerals, most of which are derived from food. When these precursor or building-block nutrients are lacking, the neurotransmitter system breaks down. It is known that severe malnutrition caused by anorexia nervosa or involuntary starvation not only leads to low weight and increased mortality rates but also to cognitive deficits and abnormal neurotransmitter activity. It has been found that supplementing with fish oil normalized the function of certain neurotransmitters and modified substance seeking in starving mice.

Severe or ongoing stress can do long-term damage to the reward system of the brain. The stressor may be in the form of a single traumatic event (experiencing an earthquake or witnessing a murder), intermittent or chronic stressful events (child abuse), a series of highly stressful situations (a death followed by a severe injury followed by a job loss), or an ongoing condition of unrelenting stress (living with an alcoholic or drug-addicted person) severely damage the reward system.

Staying Clean and Sober

The importance of extreme stress in relation to altered brain chemistry cannot be overstated. The physiology of the brain can be changed in response to chronic stress. The biochemical reaction to stress is normal and protective. Following day-to-day stress, it has been found that the anti-stress neurotransmitter dopamine is released by nerve cells to combat the effects of norepinephrine up to 100 times its normal resting state. But when stress is severe or prolonged, the levels of dopamine may never return to normal. And the condition of chronic stress sets the stage for the use of mood-altering substances to supplement dopamine levels.

Physical trauma, particularly to the head, can also lead to an imbalance in neurotransmitters. Richard, the brother, described earlier in this chapter, suffered head trauma at age six, and it was after that, that he began showing some of the characteristics that distinguished him from his brother James. While the head injury is non-genetic, you need to know, that most recently it was found that carriers of the A1 form of the DRD2 gene who have head injury show a delayed return to normal levels of cognition by at least one year.

Exposure to environmental toxins such as pesticides and heavy metals can alter brain chemistry. While there is little research on the role of heavy metals and subsequent drug-seeking behaviors, many clinicians embrace the anecdotal belief of its importance in addiction medicine. It is known that mercury toxicity diminishes the protective effect of fish and omega-3 fatty acids. And that omega-3 fatty acids increase dopamine D2 receptors in humans. Moreover, mercury inactivates the main enzyme (catecholamine-0-methyl transferase) involved in neurotransmitter breakdown. This inactivation can lead to over-expression of dopamine in the brain. As we stated earlier, too much of a good thing may be toxic. Over-expression of dopamine in certain brain regions can lead to psychosis and drug-seeking behavior to cope with it. Also, as far back as 1975, some rat data support the proposition that lead, imbibed at a critical stage of development via the lactating mother, increases the potency of morphine reinforcement as a result of changes in cerebral dopaminergic activity. In simple terms, this finding also supports anecdotal evidence that heavy metal toxicity is linked to subsequent drug abuse.

Heavy or long-term use of mood-altering substances can alter brain chemistry. So people who may not have the genetic predisposition or are not malnourished or traumatized may develop reward deficiency just by their continued use of mood-altering substances. If James had used drugs long enough and heavily enough, he might have altered his brain chemistry as well. This is important when considering the question of who becomes addicted and who doesn't.

For the most part, as we discussed earlier, people who become addicted have a genetic predisposition to it. But that doesn't mean that someone without the genetic predisposition *cannot* become addicted. Whether or not an individual becomes addicted to a substance depends upon the addictiveness of the substance, the frequency and quantity of use, and the susceptibility of the person.

Some substances are addictive to almost anyone who uses them. Nicotine is a good example. The majority of people who smoke tobacco for any length of time become addicted and find it very difficult to quit. It should be noted, however, that some people who smoke can have an easier time quitting than others. They do not smoke heavily, and when they decide to stop, they throw away their cigarettes and never pick them up again. These people cannot understand why others cannot do the same. For most people, however, smoking is highly addictive. Some individuals start smoking at a younger age and find it so difficult to quit that repeated efforts prove futile. This is most likely caused by having genetic and environmental (epigenetic) influences. There is a plethora of information linking nicotine withdrawal and potential ease in quitting to particular gene variants mostly related to dopamine function.[12]

Can we Become Addicted to Behaviors?

The process of addiction as we have described it can result from excessive consumption of substances such as alcohol, cocaine, heroin, marijuana, nicotine, sugar, or any number of prescription drugs. The same process can occur as a result of excessive behaviors or activities.

Behaviors that can become excessive and compulsive, and therefore addictions, include gambling or risk-taking, "work-aholism," excessive sexual activity, compulsive spending, and certain eating behaviors. They can also include a relationship that becomes obsessive or compulsive, playing computer games, racing cars, golfing, or running. It is not so much what you do as how you do it. You may wonder how an activity can change brain chemistry if nothing is ingested to bind to the receptor sites as a mood-altering substance does. Remember that both genes and environment play important roles in why people abuse drugs or participate in risky behaviors. With neuroimaging, we are able to see how specific brain regions respond when exposed to either psychoactive drugs or risky behaviors.

All our thoughts, feelings, and actions affect brain chemistry; and brain chemistry affects our thoughts, feelings, and actions. You have no doubt heard about the power of positive thinking. There is also power in negative thinking. Happy thoughts, as well as angry, sad, or worrying thoughts, cause a release of chemicals in the body. Were you ever in physical or emotional pain and then smiled because of something cute your child or pet did and then realized that your pain was diminished? Were you ever feeling great and then happened to think about some disturbing situation that caused you to feel tired or perhaps develop a headache? These are examples of the power of our thoughts and feelings. Research shows that a full body laugh changes your brain chemistry for up to forty-five minutes. We refer to these as endogenous chemical messengers because the release is not triggered by something you consume; it comes from within.

There are activities that change our biochemistry so much that we want to do them over and over. Some people get a biochemical response from shoplifting or inappropriate sex that is equal to or greater than the response to a heroin injection. People born with the inability to feel good will look for ways to stimulate the release of dopamine. It can happen without drugs and take the form of video games, shoplifting, gambling, inappropriate sex, all working through the brain reward circuitry to yield enough dopamine release to make us feel good from within.

And if the person has a reward deficit that predisposes to addiction, the activity that works will be repeated as often as necessary to get the desired reward. For the person predisposed to addiction, the chosen activity will rapidly proceed from self-medication to addiction.[13]

A Story of Gambling and Risk-taking Addiction

Curt developed an addiction to casino gambling. His family and friends were quite astonished by this behavior because even gambling on cards was not customary for him. A friend talked him into going to the casino the first time where he discovered a game that was a combination of skill and luck, and the challenge of it hooked him immediately. He won and it was exhilarating. He went back the next night—and the next. It He found himself thinking about and anticipating the next time he could go.

Before long, Curt was leaving work during the day and neglecting his business. He was on a winning streak, and his euphoria was beyond anything he had ever experienced with any kind of substance. When he began losing, he was sure that the next time he would make it back. It was not until his wife threatened to leave him that he went to Gamblers Anonymous and with a great struggle gave up the casino. The craving was intense. He soon satisfied this craving with cars. He started buying cars, fast cars, and driving them 120 miles an hour. In the state where he lived, this is a felony and he found himself in trouble with the law. That is when he realized that he had not stopped gambling; it had just taken another form.

Whether reward deficiency is caused by genetic or environmental factors or both, it puts individuals at higher risk for using a substance or behavior to relieve the discomfort of the deficiency and also for becoming addicted to that substance or behavior. When there is too much dopamine, it can lead to schizophrenia and when there is too little dopamine it can result in reward deficiency. So to promote a "Happy Brain," we need to ensure proper dopamine function. By intervening with solutions that provide just the right amount of dopamine synthesis and or an increase in the number of dopamine receptors, we can create dopamine homeostasis. Let's look now at what happens when those with reward deficiency syndrome discover a substance that provides what they are missing.

Thanks to Dr. Kenneth Blum for his extensive contributions to this chapter.

Three

SELF-MEDICATING REWARD DEFICIENCY

When the normal process of the reward cascade is disrupted, the resulting state of discomfort can lead to self-medicating with mood-altering substances for relief. If there is an imbalance in the reward cascade, leading to a deficiency of natural dopamine, the newly found substance (whether it's a drug, a food, or behavior) becomes a substitute for the natural chemical and, temporarily at least, corrects the deficiency. Suddenly, the anxiety, restlessness, emptiness, and cravings are gone. But over time, the good feelings are offset by the negative consequences of using the substance or behavior.

When first using a mood-altering substance or behavior, the reward-deficient person usually feels relieved, *normal* for the first time in his or her life mood-altering substances either fit the same receptors as neurotransmitters or (in the case of cocaine) cause dopamine release and also prevent the breakdown of recently released dopamine. It is well-known through much research that all abusable drugs such as methadone, morphine, heroin, amphetamines, cocaine, cannabis, nicotine, food (glucose) and risky behavioral activities like gambling or sex release different amounts of dopamine across the brain, especially at the reward site (accumbens). By consuming these substances or participating in certain behaviors, individuals are self-medicating their dopamine deficiency by stimulating dopamine receptors.

Early Use

Are individuals with reward deficiency syndrome more likely than the average person to continue using a mood-altering substance once they have found one that works for them? Of course they are. It is highly unlikely that, having discovered a way to instantly feel better, they will not do it over and over again. That is the reward they have been missing. And just as a hungry person seeks the reward of food, reward-deficient people seek what will satisfy their hunger. And the reward is immediate. They don't have to wait for a payoff. It works, it works now, and it works every time (at least in the beginning). It relieves their discomfort and gives them pleasure. They are no longer reward deficient. They have discovered a way to feel good.

It is very difficult to detect addiction in its early stages because using the substance is more beneficial than harmful for the people who are most susceptible. It provides what their brains normally lack. Just as Ritalin (a mood-altering, amphetamine-like substance) can allow some children with ADHD (a reward-deficiency condition) to function better, other drugs are beneficial for other reward-deficiency conditions. These drugs may make it possible to be more sociable, more at ease, and demonstrate a higher level of social skills. Physical performance may even improve.

Contrary to the common belief that consuming increasing quantities of alcohol results in a decreased ability to function, people may actually perform some tasks better when they are somewhat intoxicated. This is due in part to "inate tolerance." This means that they (compared to individuals who are not at risk for addiction), have more ability to handle the first hit of alcohol or other psychoactive drug, and they even recover faster from the "high."

In 1982, in three different genetically inbred strains of mice having different "likes" for alcohol (some loved it, some were indifferent, and some hated it), it was found that the mice that loved alcohol were less sensitive and able to recover more rapidly from the effects of the same dose of alcohol than the other two strains. This "inate tolerance" was also observed in humans almost a decade later.

Consequently, the earliest warning sign of the onset of addiction (the ability to function well), interferes with early diagnosis and makes it difficult for a developing addict or others to recognize there is a problem. The ability to "hold their liquor" (or nicotine or marijuana or prescription drug) actually conceals the problem and creates the belief among early stage addicts that they are immune to the painful consequences that they see others experience because of drinking or drug use. Addiction is a disease that appears to be beneficial in the early stage, allowing the person to experience the rewarding effects without paying any of the penalties.

Remember Andrea from the previous chapter? She knew from the first drink that she would continue to use alcohol to feel good. She knew immediately that it took away all the things about her that always made her feel different. At first she could drink with no problems. She could drink more than her friends could without getting drunk. She was able to function better after she had a few drinks than she could sober. She felt more free to express herself. She started writing poetry and thought she had found or released her creative side.

Merlene Miller, MA and David Miller, PhD

Continued Use and Tolerance

All the while, however, the brain is changing and adapting to the regular ingestion of the drug. Early on, these changes may seem beneficial. People who are becoming addicted can usually tolerate larger and larger quantities without becoming intoxicated and without experiencing harmful consequences, just like the alcohol-loving mice. But over time, continued heavy use, especially by people with a genetic predisposition and/or poor environment, leads to addiction. As they are able to consume increasing quantities and their bodies adapt to the presence of these larger quantities, they eventually *must* use even larger quantities to get the same effect, creating more and more changes in the brain.

Andrea found that as she drank more, she was able to drink even more. She began to find that the amounts she had used before no longer did for her what they used to, and she increased the frequency and quantity of her drinking. She was unaware that biochemical and physical changes were taking place in her brain which were setting her up for problems. She thought she was in no danger of becoming addicted because she could "hold her liquor" better than anyone she knew. She was not aware that this was an early warning sign of alcoholism. Alcohol was her best friend and, she thought, her friend for life.

Using Addictive Substances to Relieve the Painful Consequences of Using Addictive Substances

When substance use is heavy and continual, the good feelings produced at first are eventually negated by the painful consequences.

These consequences can come in many forms. Problems may arise from drinking and driving or other violations of the law. There may be family or job problems. Or there may be physical complications. Whatever the problems are, the user now knows how to make the pain go away. Using the mood-altering substance temporarily takes away pain. So the person, now feeling some painful consequences, uses more and more. The more pain, the more use. The need to use the substance to relieve the pain of using the substance blocks the awareness of what is really causing the pain.

What is happening in the brain at this point is that the mood-altering substance is interfering with the release of neurotransmitters and blocking the receptors. With heavier use, fewer neurotransmitters are being produced and released. And it takes more and more of the substance to fill the receptors and get high.

Let's get back to Andrea. To her surprise, she began to have problems because of her drinking. At first, she did not realize that these problems had anything to do with drinking. She began skipping school and thought she was just having a good time. When she was caught and punished at home and suspended from school, she told herself that everyone was just overreacting to her free spirit. She felt misunderstood and angry. What did she do? She drank more in order to get the comfort of dopamine.

Dependence

When a substance is used regularly, it shuts down the release of dopamine from the neuron. This is further complicated by blocking the effects of other important proteins responsible for breaking down or clearing dopamine from the synapse. So too much of the substance can lead to a reduction in the production of dopamine, less dopamine released from the neuron, (causing less dopamine in the synapse) and reduction in number of dopamine receptors needed for dopamine to act on the brain. The outcome is what we term "hypodopaminergic" or low dopamine.

Addicts are unaware that physiological and biochemical changes are occurring as long as they are able to drink or get their drug. They think they are functioning normally. And they may believe they are drinking or using responsibly or at least attempting to do so. When enough problems occur, addicts may attempt to control their use. But by the time they are aware that their alcohol or other drug use is the problem, they cannot choose to use responsibly. As the brain adapts to higher levels of the substance, the body accepts this as normal and demands that this new state of normal be maintained.

While tolerance is increasing, so is dependence. Craving for the substance leads to continued substance use despite the painful consequences. The person cannot function without the substance. The person no longer uses the substance to simply feel good or to relieve the painful consequences caused by the substance. As neurons in the brain adapt to larger and larger quantities, many changes occur at important regions of the brain involved with inducing pleasure and reducing stress. When the brain does not get its supply from an outside source, it does not snap into production and start supplying the needed chemicals. It screams out for more dopamine. The addict now uses alcohol or other drugs only to relieve the painful consequences of *not* using them. This is when the survival (craving) part of the brain takes over. It believes it must have the substance to survive. It overpowers the rational (judgment) part of the brain, and obtaining the substance becomes as strong and vital a need as breathing. Noted journalist Bill Moyers has called this the "hijacked brain." The drug has essentially stolen the addict's ability to think rationally and to choose responsibly.

When Andrea got married, her husband objected to her heavy drinking, so she decided she would cut back. But her attempts were short lived. She would cut back for a few days and then soon find that she was back to her regular amount. As this became more and more of a problem in her marriage, she tried many ways to drink in moderation. She would set rules—then break them. She would promise herself she would only drink during certain times of the day. Or that she would drink only on weekends. Or that she would only drink beer. Or that she would drink only with other people. But she broke every promise she made to her husband and herself. Fearing her husband was going to leave her, Jan promised to quit entirely. And she did. For two days. She was sick and miserable for those two days. She never stopped thinking about drinking. She was obsessed with the idea of having just one. The compulsion to take that one drink was overpowering. Finally, convinced she could have one and stop, she gave in and soon her drinking was out of control again. Not surprisingly, her husband did leave her which provided her a real reason to drink, and alcohol completely took over her life.

The Pleasure Is Gone

What was once the great friend has now become an enemy. At this point the addict develops drug toxicity. The decreased release of neurotransmitters, and fewer receptors along with diminished ethanol liver enzymes (needed to clear alcohol from the body) lead the inability to hold one's liquor. The drug no longer produces any pleasure. It creates psychological and physical pain, suffering, and misery. Instead of being able to use more and more, addicts at this point can use less and less before becoming sick, out of control, afraid, and miserable.

There is pain when using drugs and pain when not using them. The drug has depleted the brain's supply of natural feel-good chemicals and the drug is no longer a satisfactory substitute. Addicts continue to use alcohol or other drugs, not for any pleasure, but only because the survival part of the brain has taken over and believes it must have the substance or die. Attempts to stop are usually short lived and futile. Severe anxiety results when an unexpected situation interferes with the substance use or the source of supply.

At this point, many of the addict's family, friends, and associates believe the person is behaving irresponsibly, unaware that the person is not choosing the behavior—that it is being dictated by the survival part of the brain. It takes less and less of the substance before the person loses control and experiences symptoms of intoxication. The person may go immediately from the pain of needing the drug to the pain of using the drug. The magic is gone. The pleasure is gone. There is nothing but pain. Pain while not using the substance. Pain while using it.

Andrea doesn't remember when the pleasure stopped and drinking brought her only pain. At first she thought she was so miserable because her husband had left her. Gradually she became aware that drinking was giving her no comfort. She was getting drunk more and more often. She could drink less and less before getting sick. Where had the magic gone? She was convinced she could find it again if she could just find the secret door. She tried to work at several jobs but was too sick most of the time to go to work. She was lonely and started going out with friends with whom she previously drank, those people who used to comment about her ability to hold her liquor. But now she was passing out and they were driving her home. They didn't like being with her any more. Every day she would promise herself that tomorrow she would stop. But tomorrow she only remade the promise.

Eventually Andrea was able to get sober with the help of Alcoholics Anonymous (AA). But it was the hardest thing she ever did, and now she lives one day at a time, recognizing that she can never learn to drink in moderation. Still she grieves the loss of her best friend, alcohol. She yearns for the comfort it gave her and is looking for something else that might give her some of the pleasure she found in drinking.

Abstinence

There are times when addicted people may have a moment of sanity and realize that if they keep using they will die. Thus, they may ask for help. They may enter a treatment center. If it is a treatment center without medical detoxification or dopamine- agonist therapy, the pain of abstinence is so severe that addicts frequently leave before they have made it all the way through the detoxification process. If they receive medical detoxification, many stick it out even though they are uncomfortable. But what happens now to the poor brain, totally depleted of natural brain chemicals and unable to produce an adequate supply? Usually nothing. It stays that way. Perhaps for months, perhaps for years. Perhaps forever. Whether due to conditions that existed before addiction or that result from addiction, it is reward deficient.

In many cases, what was discomfort prior to substance use now is even more intense. And the brain continues to crave the substance upon which it has come to depend. After struggling through months of pain, misery, and craving, many addicts give up in despair, and believing there is no way out, go back to what they know will at least relieve the craving, if not the pain.

Over a period of thirteen years, Mark, a heroin addict, attempted recovery many times (he thinks as many as fifty). Sometimes he left before he got through detox and went right back to using heroin. Sometimes he made it through a thirty-day treatment program and stayed clean for a while. Always during his periods of sobriety, he went to 12-step meetings. But he was totally depleted of energy. He says he was so lethargic that sometimes he couldn't get out of bed. He did not have the energy to work at his job in construction. Sometimes he thought he might have some kind of illness, but nothing was ever diagnosed. Finally, believing he would never be able to function normally again, he would give up and go back to heroin. No matter how hard he tried, he was never able to maintain more than thirty days of sobriety. That is, until he received treatment that provided dopamine homeostasis and provided relief from the pain of abstinence and gave him energy necessary to function normally.

Now, many people will tell you that Mark was just not motivated to get sober—that if he *really* wanted to, he could do it. But why would he go to treatment over and over again, usually voluntarily, unless he really wanted to free himself from his addiction?

Remember that he had been in treatment as many as fifty times. Why would you attempt something for the fiftieth time—you had already failed at forty-nine previous times—if you didn't really want it? Some people might say that Mark just hadn't hurt enough yet. No, it was not the lack of pain that kept him locked into his addiction. *It was too much pain.* It was not until his brain was healed and he was relieved of his pain that he was able to live a normal life. Some people will tell you that Mark just did not have any self-discipline. How many of us have the self-discipline to endure ongoing, unrelenting pain without relief—and no relief in sight—without looking for some source of pain relief?

Staying Clean and Sober

Let us be clear here that many addicted people do make it and find ways to maintain sobriety. Many find a better life through practicing the program of a 12-step group. Millions of recovering people are living proof that sobriety and recovery from addiction are possible. Through their experience of addiction and recovery they find meaning and purpose and are able to live in serenity and peace. *We are concerned for those who do not find this path.* While some do find relief from their addictions, the majority of those who are addicted do not. Their craving addictive brains interfere with their ability to follow the road that has led to recovery for others.

So, for someone experiencing the discomfort and/or pleasure deficit of imbalanced neurochemistry, mood-altering chemicals do, for a period of time, work to bring relief and feelings of pleasure and well being. But eventually the good feelings of self-medication are replaced by the pain of addiction.

What starts out as a rewarding experience—and perhaps an improvement in the ability to function—becomes a dependence on the substance in order to function. This happens as the drug further impairs the reward system of the brain and further impairs neurological functioning. The impairment may be so severe that the person is physically, emotionally, and mentally unable to function without the drug. The need to use the drug overpowers normal reasoning and previous life values.

When the addict attempts to abstain, craving for the substance to relieve the pain of impaired neurochemistry during withdrawal leads the person back to use of the substance over and over again. Therefore, relapse is common and may lead to feelings of hopelessness and the belief that sobriety is impossible. Many addicts give up and finally experience physical, economic, and social deterioration or—too frequently—death.

Attempting recovery from addiction, then, without addressing the neurological pain and craving that accompany it, is much like attempting recovery from diabetes without addressing the functioning of the pancreas. Most treatment is helpful in that it helps addicts cope with the craving and pain of abstinence, but does not take it away. With scientific information now available, more options are becoming available to re-balance brain chemistry and restore normal neurotransmission, thus relieving the craving and discomfort of abstinence. This frees the addict to focus on other necessary tasks of recovery: rebuilding a damaged and impaired life and developing a new lifestyle that will support the maintenance of healthy brain chemistry.

A Story of Addiction

Fred began drinking mouthwash when he was four or five years old. He was a restless, impulsive child. Drinking mouthwash made him feel good. When he was ten he found a bag of marijuana his father had taken from an older brother. He replaced the marijuana in the bag with parsley and smoked the marijuana. It made him feel great. From that day on he smoked marijuana daily. He knew from early childhood that mood-altering substances would be an important part of his life. But it never occurred to him that there might come a time when drugs might become an enemy rather than a friend.

Fred stayed high on marijuana or alcohol most of the time throughout his childhood. Even so, he maintained good grades with little effort. His family and teachers had no idea he was hiding such a habit. In ninth grade he began using speed (amphetamine) and crack cocaine. He was still able to function all right. He was part of a very wealthy family, so getting money for the drugs was never a problem.

Staying Clean and Sober

Fred had only good experiences with drugs until he started using a needle. He says that nothing was ever the same again. The rush from injected drugs was the most important thing in his life. By that time he was around twenty. Soon he was speed balling (using cocaine and heroin together). Daily use caused him no problems for about nine months. Then his friend very rapidly became his enemy. There was no longer pleasure from the drugs. He was sick and miserable.

Fred knew he needed to get off the heroin and cocaine, so he decided to try treatment. He stopped using heroin and cocaine (detoxed with Librium). He continued to smoke marijuana during treatment and never intended to give up marijuana and alcohol. After eighteen days he was feeling fine and decided he didn't need any more treatment and abruptly left the treatment center. Four months later he was again injecting 3.5 grams of cocaine and 3 grams of heroin daily.

At this point Fred knew he was in deep trouble and thought there was no way out. A large inheritance made it easy to keep doing what he was doing. He came to the conclusion that he was one of those people who was on earth to live fast and die young. He deteriorated rapidly. He was part of what he calls a ruthless drug scene. He was sharing needles, shooting up crack. It didn't take long to go through his inheritance.

He tried working for his brother for awhile. But it was physical labor, and he was in bad physical condition. He was 6'2" yet weighed only 155 pounds. He was weak and sweating within a half-hour of beginning work. But he had to wear long sleeves to cover the needle marks. He was always late and took bathroom breaks every twenty minutes. So much for trying to work.

By the time Fred had been injecting drugs seven years he says he found it quite ironic that his mother was a millionaire and he had turned into a bum. "I could have had anything I wanted, but I didn't want anything but drugs." He was living in his truck, shooting up while driving. He was getting no pleasure from the drugs; he was just trying to stay alive and truly believed he would die without them. At the same time he knew he was going to die if he kept on the road he was on. Six of his friends had died within the previous year. He thought there was no way out. No hope. Just waiting to die.

Periodically Fred would see his mother to get money. One day she was crying and told him she knew what he was doing. He told her he didn't know any other way to live. She told him of a treatment she had heard about that might work for him. She begged him to try. He agreed to go after the holidays. Four hours later he was sitting in jail. He had been stopped by the police with needles and spoons all over his truck. Though drugs were hidden in his socks, they weren't found so he was charged with nineteen misdemeanors but no felonies. His mother posted bond and took him directly to treatment where, very near death, he received some of the therapies we will discuss in later chapters.

Integrating what he learned in treatment into his life, Fred has found that his intense craving for drugs has disappeared. He has continued to take the nutrients he received in treatment. He attends 12-step meetings, and he has started college. He enjoys surfing and playing basketball and just being physically active. After several months he says he can think about drugs without craving them. He feels no need for substitute drugs. Fred feels that he has a real life, something he thought he could never have. He says he has goals — which he never had before. At age twenty-seven, he feels he has just been born.

Four

The Pain of Ineffective Treatment and Relapse

Addiction to alcohol and other drugs takes its toll on the lives of those who are addicted and their families and on society as a whole. It kills by overdose, by accidents, by suicides, by homicides, by destroying the mind and body, and by causing other diseases that disable and kill. It tears apart families, fills our prisons, steals our children, and drains our economy. Consider the following:[1]

- Our nation's drug problem costs $193 billion per year. This figure includes legal, medical, and treatment costs; the cost of lost productivity on the job; the cost of drug-related crime; and the cost of social programs that address poverty, child and spouse abuse and other social issues that result directly and indirectly from addiction.
- More than 1 in 7 Americans ages 12 and older have a drug or alcohol problem.

- Of the 2.3 million inmates in this country's prisons and jails, 85% are there for drug-related crimes.
- Including those under probation or parole, nearly 7 million adults are involved with the criminal justice system.
- Alcohol and other drugs are associated with child abuse, rapes, assaults, suicides, spousal abuse, traffic fatalities, murders, and drowning.
- Alcohol and other drug use is the overall leading cause of death in the United States.

We know you are thinking that we are wrong about the last statement because drug and alcohol use is listed by the government behind cancer and heart disease as a leading cause of death. But cancer death rates *include* lung cancer deaths due to nicotine addiction and pancreatic and liver cancer deaths due to alcoholism. Heart disease death rates include deaths from heart problems due to heroin and cocaine addiction. Diabetes death rates include deaths from complications of alcoholism. Adding homicides, suicides, and accidents attributable to alcohol and drug use, it can easily be seen that alcohol and other drug use is *the* leading cause of death in the nation.

Yet while progress has been made in the treatment of cancer, heart disease, and diabetes, little has been done to change the dismal rates of recovery from addiction, whether addiction to alcohol, nicotine, illegal drugs, or prescription drugs. Little or no progress has been made in the effectiveness of treatment for alcoholism and other drug addictions in the last forty years. Although there are not consistent and accurate methods of attaining addiction recovery and relapse rates, statistics indicate that the recovery rate has not changed much in the last forty years and claims less than a 20 percent success rate. However, there is no health problem more serious or more widespread.

Is Lack of Treatment the Problem?

Lack of available treatment is often blamed for the cost of addiction to individuals and to society. And it is true—there is a shortage of treatment. From treatment professionals, from those pushing for treatment rather than incarceration, and from those wanting more tax dollars we often hear the phrase "treatment works." *But if available treatment is effective for only a small percentage of the people who get it, then we need more than additional treatment; we need better, more effective, treatment.* In the treatment of addiction, we are doing the same thing over and over, trying for a different result rather than looking for better answers. If you always do what you always did, you'll always get what you always got.

Although there is a scarcity of treatment, this is not the major reason for the severe problems related to addiction in the United States. *Relapse* is the major reason for the high rate of social, medical, and personal problems associated with addiction. Most people who enter conventional treatment centers will relapse, usually more than once, often repeatedly. Effective treatment would reduce relapse rates and improve the quality of sobriety as well as reduce the destruction that results from addiction.

There is little understanding of addiction or how to treat it by those who most often encounter it: health professionals, human service workers, and those in the criminal justice system. Courses in addiction are seldom taught in medical schools, nursing schools, or schools of theology. Nor are they taught in psychology, social work, or criminal justice programs in colleges and universities. Addiction professionals often don't have a college degree, and they draw largely from their own experience or from what has been done in the past (with a recovery rate of less than 20 percent).

While acknowledging that addiction is truly a physical disease—with profound psychological and social consequences—addiction professionals have primarily addressed the *consequences,* directing little treatment toward the physical disease itself or its underlying causes. Most addiction professionals have recognized that it is a disease, but many don't really understand *how* it is a disease or how it comes about; therefore, they don't know how to treat the condition directly. Consequently, the main goal of conventional treatment has been to teach people how to accept and cope with *symptoms.*

On the other hand, there are a few treatment centers that do focus on physical recovery, most of which, unfortunately, do not emphasize the other aspects of wellness. Addiction is a physical condition with psychological, behavioral, social, and spiritual consequences. The first step is to treat the unhealthy neurochemistry and physiology of the brain, but treatment that ends there is incomplete. The addict is left with life deficits that cannot be overcome by fixing the brain alone. Even more of a problem is the growing tendency by health professionals to treat addiction with prescription (often mood-altering) medications. Even when used along with counseling and support groups, this practice does not improve recovery rates.

Symptoms that Interfere With the Ability to Stay Sober

Perhaps what is least understood about the nature of addiction is that there are painful symptoms that occur during abstinence that interfere with the ability to stay sober: craving, stress sensitivity, anxiety, dysphoria, depression, mental confusion, inability to concentrate, increased pain sensitivity, sleep disturbances, and hypersensitivity to the environment.[2]

Most people are unaware that the pain of staying sober can be, and frequently is, so severe that it interferes with the ability to function even when the desire for and commitment to recovery is strong. This chronic discomfort is what leads to relapse.

Most addiction treatment is beneficial in the limited sense that it teaches coping skills for living with the craving and the pain of abstinence. But it does not take them away. While this approach helps many people stay sober, for the majority, those with severe symptoms (which we will discuss in more detail later in this chapter), it is not enough. Some hang on; some find substitute addictions; most relapse. Two out of three addicts who enter treatment will relapse, usually within the first three to four months. Some who struggle unsuccessfully may go through treatment twenty—even fifty—times. (Unfortunately, after a couple of failures, they may be refused admittance to some treatment centers.) Their desire to maintain sobriety is strong, so strong that they keep trying over and over again, even after repeated unsuccessful attempts.

While scientific research has opened doors to new understanding of the nature of addiction and its effect on the brain, medical and addiction professionals have applied little of this information to actually helping people get well from this devastating disease. There is a gap between what is known about addiction and what is done about it.

The Contribution of Alcoholics Anonymous[2]

Before Alcoholics Anonymous (AA) was started in the 1930s alcoholism was considered a hopeless condition. Rarely did anyone recover. Bill Wilson certainly seemed hopeless. He had tried all the cures available, but sobriety always eluded him. After an experience he called a "spiritual awakening" and involvement in the

Oxford Group where he became acquainted with and began to practice some principles for spiritual living, he was able to get a foothold on sobriety. But when he was sent to Akron, Ohio, on an extended business trip, he found himself craving alcohol and sorely tempted to take a drink. Instead, he asked around to find another alcoholic and was directed to a physician, Dr. Bob, who was receptive to the message of the Oxford Group. By sharing his story, Bill was able to avoid a return to drinking, and the fellowship of Bill and Bob was the beginning of the fellowship of Alcoholics Anonymous (AA).

In the years since, AA has spread all over the world and has become the means of recovery for thousands and thousands of alcoholics. The program has been applied to other addictions in the form of Narcotics Anonymous, Overeaters Anonymous, Smokers Anonymous, Sexual Addicts Anonymous, Gamblers Anonymous, and many more.

What does AA offer that has enabled so many people to become sober when they otherwise couldn't? For some it is simply the fellowship, having others available that have walked the same path and are willing and available to help. For some, it's working the twelve steps, which include acceptance of powerlessness over alcohol, willingness to accept help from a higher power, acknowledging and admitting character defects, making amends for wrongdoings, taking regular moral inventory, promptly admitting wrongs, maintaining contact with a higher power through prayer and meditation, and carrying the message of AA to others. For many it is the combination of this change of life focus and the support of other recovering people that provides the strength to put one foot in front of the other until the road becomes smoother.

The 12 Steps of Alcoholics Anonymous

1. We admitted we were powerless over alcohol, that our lives had become unmanageable.
2. Came to believe that a power greater than ourselves could restore us to sanity.
3. Made a decision to turn our will and our lives over to the care of God as we understood Him.
4. Made a searching and fearless moral inventory of ourselves.
5. Admitted to God, to ourselves, and to another human being the exact nature of our wrongs.
6. Were entirely ready to have God remove all these defects of character.
7. Humbly asked Him to remove our shortcomings.
8. Made a list of all persons we had harmed and became willing to make amends to them all.
9. Made direct amends to such people wherever possible, except when to do so would injure them or others.
10. Continued to take personal inventory and when we were wrong promptly admitted it.
11. Sought through prayer and meditation to improve our conscious contact with God, as we understood Him, praying only for knowledge of His will for us and the power to carry that out.
12. Having had a spiritual awakening as the result of these steps, we tried to carry this message to alcoholics, and to practice these principles in all our affairs.

Merlene Miller, MA and David Miller, PhD

The Disease Model of Addiction[3]

From its earliest days, Alcoholics Anonymous has embraced the concept that some people are able to drink alcohol without becoming addicted while others are not; and those unable to control what happens when they drink must remain abstinent. This is the underlying concept that is referred to as the "disease model" of addiction and is the basis of traditional treatment.

There are several hallmarks of the disease model of alcoholism. The first, as we have just stated, is that the distinction between social drinking and alcoholism lies in the person, not in the substance. Originally it was not known what it was within individuals that set them apart, but it has always been assumed that it was biological rather than psychological. It has sometimes been called an allergy, and while it is not, it is comparable. Most people can eat and enjoy peanuts with no problem. A few people experience a dangerous reaction to peanuts (hives, difficulty breathing, severe swelling, loss of consciousness) that can even be life threatening. The difference lies in the biological makeup of the people eating the peanuts.

Another basic tenet of the disease model is that once a person has become an alcoholic that person can never learn to drink in moderation; therefore total abstinence is necessary. The preponderance of the evidence shows this to be true.

Yet, while recognizing addiction as a physiological, biochemical abnormality rather than a psychological problem, the disease model of treatment has consisted mainly of strategies for changing beliefs, attitudes, thinking, behavior, and spiritual principles. This enables people to cope with the disease, but does not change physiology or biochemistry. These principles have proved effective for thousands of people and enabled many to stay sober who otherwise could not. Without these contributions, attitudes toward addiction and treatment might have remained in the dark ages and in the same category as bloodletting. While research has found that there is a change in brain chemistry with thinking, behavior, and spiritual principles, Primarily these are principles for living, not treatment for a disease, and they do not address the underlying neurochemical condition that accompanies addiction. They are methods of coping with the condition, not treating it.

This psychological, social, and spiritual approach to interrupting active addiction works for less than 20 percent of those who receive it. And, understandably, *those 20 percent become the spokespersons for this approach to recovery.* The belief that it is effective for anyone who truly wants to recover and who works the program has become the underpinning for addiction treatment as most people know it. There is an abundance of treatment programs built upon this foundation. The scarcity lies in the availability of treatment for the 80 percent who do not recover and are then blamed for their own failure. These relapsers believe what they have been told by the 20 percent—that the failure lies in them, not in the treatment. *We speak for this silent majority.*

For the 80% who relapse, working the conventional program has not enabled them to maintain sobriety. And many, while abstinent, have lived lives of quiet agony, never able to find comfort without the drug that once had provided it. For them, pain accompanies the choice to stop using the substance—during the period of acute withdrawal symptoms and for months and years even decades into sobriety.

A word from David: When I first made a sincere commitment to quit drinking, I tried a variety of things to help me. I found that I could not do it with will power, no matter how I tried. I went through an outpatient program at the VA hospital where

I got Mellaril (a powerful mood-altering prescription medication) and ping-pong therapy. Not very successful. Not successful at all. I finally agreed to go to an Alcoholics Anonymous meeting. Everyone there was older than I was, and I didn't identify with their war stories. So I didn't go back—until I was in danger of losing my family and realized nothing else was working. I went back with a different attitude. And after a few relapses was able to stay sober. I remember how proud I was when I was recognized at AA for one year of sobriety. What a milestone. But it was a tough year. Even with all the help I had from my AA family I struggled with stress sensitivity, emotional overreaction, cravings, and—long before I had a name for it or a way to describe it—stimulus augmentation.

With Merlene's help I found many ways of coping one day at a time. Nutrition, exercise, plenty of sleep, escape time, and participation in a church community all helped me hang on and work the program of AA. It was years later, when I started taking an amino acid supplement, developed by Kenneth Blum, that I found real relief from chronic abstinence symptoms. I am thankful for the freedom that amino acid therapy brought into my life. I will be forever grateful to AA because without it I would never have made it to that point. But I understand the pain that leads people back to drinking or using drugs when AA is not enough to heal the broken brain.

Chronic Abstinence Symptoms[4]

There are painful symptoms of addiction that occur when someone is using, symptoms that motivate the person to give up addictive use. When the pain becomes severe enough, addicted people usually choose recovery. Recovery requires abstinence, but abstinence triggers new symptoms—or the return of old symptoms that preceded the addiction. Some symptoms pass within a few days, but some emerge and grow more severe as acute withdrawal symptoms subside. Long-term and excessive use of addictive substances causes nutrient depletion and tissue and cellular damage that create reward deficiency or intensify the problems of reward deficiency that existed before addictive use began. So when addictive use stops, the symptoms that led to self-medicating with a mood-altering substance return with greater intensity.

The pain of abstinence usually takes the form of severe anxiety or depression, trouble concentrating and remembering, inability to manage stress, sleep problems, lack of energy, overwhelming cravings, and heightened sensitivity to sights, sounds, touch, and pain.

STIMULUS AUGMENTATION

This is one term used to describe heightened sensitivity to external and internal stimuli. Sometimes it is referred to as hyper-augmentation, hypersensitivity, or simply augmentation. People with this condition are unable to filter out background noises and happenings and feel bombarded by all that is going on around them. They augment or magnify sounds, sights, touch, pain, perceptions, and stress. They feel constantly overwhelmed by everything going on around them and everything going on inside them. What would usually be considered mild stress is major stress. Sounds that others do not notice are major distractions. Pain is more intense. Being touched can sometimes feel like being mauled. People with this condition feel overwhelmed by an overwhelming world.

In most cases this symptom is genetic. Alcoholics, children of alcoholics, and those with ADHD have all been found to magnify perceptual input and this has been associated with craving for alcohol. Stimulus augmentation exists prior to addiction and probably contributes to the risk that someone will use mood- altering substances at an early age. Alcohol and other drugs normalize this condition. But with abstinence it returns in full force.

INABILITY TO CONCENTRATE
An inability to concentrate is a natural result of stimulus augmentation. When the buzzing of a fly demands as much attention as the person talking to you, it is difficult to stay focused on what that person is saying. It is not rudeness; it is not intentional. It is just very difficult to maintain focus when everything around you is calling to you at the same time with the same urgency. It can be frustrating and embarrassing to realize that someone is talking to you and you have no idea what they just said.

MEMORY PROBLEMS
Memory problems result from the inability to concentrate. If you didn't hear it or were distracted when it occurred, you won't remember it, or the memory will be sketchy. You can't recall what was never really recorded in your brain in the first place. All memory problems are not the result of being unable to concentrate. Impaired memory is inherent in the neurotrasmitter deficits that accompany addiction. Normally parts of the brain talk to each. So the survival or craving part of the brain talks to the decision–making part of the brain and, in turn, to the memory part of the brain. This is called resting state functional connectivity, which is impaired by addiction. But if the brain is not connecting these important areas of the brain, memory problems can develop.

ANXIETY

Anxiety is common during recovery. Of course a certain amount of psychological stress is expected because of so much change going on. Change is stressful, and it is normal to have some fear connected with all the changes necessary to make recovery possible. But stress is exacerbated to the point of anxiety by stimulus augmentation, the inability to concentrate, memory problems, and imbalanced brain chemistry.

DYSPHORIA

This is a general feeling of discomfort or unpleasantness. It is the absence of pleasure from doing things that would normally be pleasurable. It can range from mild to severe and is characterized by listlessness, lack of motivation and, sometimes, hopelessness. Ongoing dysphoria takes the color out of life and puts sobriety in jeopardy. Sometimes the dysphoria comes and goes and takes the form of mood swings. Sometimes you feel good and then soon feel very down. The tendency for you and the people around you is to believe when you are feeling good that you are always going to feel good; it is then quite disheartening when you are again overcome by dysphoria.

DRUG HUNGER (CRAVING)

Intense craving, or what some refer to as drug hunger, is a powerful compulsion to alter one's mood with a psychoactive drug. As we explained in chapter two, people with reward deficiency lack adequate dopamine to provide the satisfaction that other people get from normal activities. They crave something more just to feel normal. Feeling incomplete or inadequate or unfulfilled is common with abstinence. There is a feeling of emptiness and a yearning for something—anything—to fill up the emptiness. The emptiness begs for self-medication. The sober person experiencing cravings knows what will bring relief.

To evaluate the severity of your abstinence symptoms, rate each of the following symptoms from 0 – 10 with 0 representing the absence of the symptom and 10 repensenting an extreme intensity level. You can use this to measure the severity of the symptoms you are experiencing at any time. This is helpful to determine how effective any strategy you are trying is. Rate each symptom 1-10 in severity. Test yourself now and when you begin a new therapy. When you begin any of the therapies in this book, rate your symptoms each day to see how well you are doing. This rating scale will also help you to determine when your symptoms are getting worse, indicating that you need may be heading for relapse and need more help than you are getting.

1. Craving or drug huger _____5_____
2. Sense of emptiness or incompleteness _____3_____
3. Anxiety _____0_____
4. Internal shakiness _____0_____
5. Impulsivity _____0_____
6. Difficulty concentrating _____5_____
7. Memory problems _____8_____
8. Depression _____5_____
9. Irritability _____0_____
10. Restlessness _____0_____
11. Problems getting to or staying asleep _____5_____
12. Fatigue/lack of energy _____5_____
13. Hypersensitivity to stress _____0_____
14. Hypersensitivity to noise, sights, or touch _____0_____
15. Hypersensitivity to pain _____0_____

Total Score _____36_____

The Stress of Sobriety

Stress intensifies all the symptoms of abstinence. When you make a commitment to sobriety, everything in your life changes, and change is always stressful. And dealing daily with stimulus augmentation, the inability to concentrate, memory problems, mood swings, and cravings creates additional stress.

In handling stress the brain uses large quantities of neurochemicals. Persistent, ongoing stress not only raises the level of stress hormones, but depletes the brain of key neurochemicals that relieve stress. So during recovery when you are expected to be getting better, the stress of abstinence may actually make you feel worse. People tell you to just hang on and things will get better, but they don't. The daily stress of maintaining abstinence (plus the high levels of stress hormones) may be further depleting your neurotransmitter stores. During times of stress the body releases chemicals to help us keep functioning, but the constant excess of these chemicals can cause irritability, sleeplessness, depression, anxiety, and eventually physical illnesses (high blood pressure, heart disease, and gastrointestinal problems, to mention a few), all of which become new stressors.

Constitutionally Incapable of Rigorous Honesty

While it offers hope, the book of Alcoholics Anonymous (referred to as The Big Book[5]) does state that there are those for whom the program doesn't work. It says this is not their fault because they are "constitutionally incapable of being rigorously honest." Well, why would some be *constitutionally* incapable of being rigorously honest and why would that interfere with a sincere effort to maintain sobriety?

The answer lies in what we call denial. Denial is a mechanism we employ to protect us from a truth too painful to face. For many addicts the truth of what it takes to maintain abstinence is something too uncomfortable to tolerate. The program of AA requires a person to look squarely at themselves. But for those "constitutionally" incapable of being rigorously honest, denial becomes a wall that will not allow them to look into themselves for fear of the truth they will find. In many people the pain of abstinence becomes so severe that it blocks the ability to do the work of recovery. Sometimes we hear that pain is the great motivator and that is true. Pain *does* motivate us to do whatever we need to do to get rid of it. It does *not* motivate us to do what will create more pain. And, when the pain of abstinence is severe and doesn't let up, it is not a motivation to stick with the painful tasks required. Rather, it interferes with the ability to do so.

Consider for a moment a time when you had some other severe pain. Now consider your reaction if someone were to ask you, at the point of this severe pain, to take a piece of paper and write down your character defects. How capable would you be of doing that while experiencing this pain? But supposing you were somehow able to do that, and, after you did it, you were given another piece of paper and asked to make a list of all the people you have harmed in your life and to state what you are willing to do to make amends to these people. You would probably be constitutionally incapable of doing that. But in some drug treatment programs this is exactly what you are asked to do. *For some people, it is the pain of abstinence that renders them "constitutionally incapable of being rigorously honest."*

Sobriety: Is It Really This Difficult?

I've been sober for a few months, but my brain just feels numb—I don't know how to think or what to think or even if I want to think.

I haven't had a drink in seven weeks, but I feel like I'm going nuts. When my kids yell at each other, I want to curl up into a ball and die. Bright lights, loud noises, intense emotions—I can't be around them. I feel like they are frying my brain.

I'm sober, but my memory is shot, and I'm afraid I have permanent brain damage or maybe even Alzheimer's.

I can't figure it out. I've got eight months of sobriety under my belt, but the anxiety and the fear just don't quit. Once or twice a week I wake up in a sweat, dreaming about the time I ran over my son's bicycle when I was drunk and imagining that I killed him.

Some days I feel great, happy, solidly sober, but then the next day I feel just plain awful. My mood swings are like flash floods—there's never any warning.

I cry all the time. I'm always overreacting to everything—a pile of dirty clothes in the hallway is enough to make me want to scream.

I'm telling you—alcoholism was hell. But what is this, purgatory?

From *Beyond the Influence*[5]

These symptoms persist even with participation in recovery activities; and deep inside, the addicted person is always aware of what will provide pain relief. While some people hang on in spite of the discomfort, "white knuckling" it through life, many cannot and eventually give in to the compulsion to drink or take other drugs or to develop a substitute addiction such as gambling or a food addiction.

There is currently enough scientific information about the biochemical nature of addiction to go beyond treatment methods commonly available. Traditional psychological, spiritual, and behavioral methods are helpful and should not be discarded, but it is time for a marriage between these methods and new strategies based on scientific information available. It is time to close the gap between what we know and what we do to heal the addicted brain. And that is why we have written this book--to help you do that.

Five

THOSE AMAZING AMINOS

In our search for lasting and effective treatment for addiction, by far the most remarkable discovery so far has been amino acid therapy. Neurotransmitters are made from amino acids, the building blocks of protein. Several key neurotransmitters are particularly affected by and involved in addiction. These neurochemicals need to be balanced to their normal state in order for the recovering person to be free of chronic abstinence symptoms such as cravings, anxiety, irritability, and depression. Over the past thirty years, numerous addiction clinicians have begun treating the brain with certain amino acids that can help restore healthy brain chemistry. This treatment is based on over 30 published clinical trials.[1]

In this book we will sometimes refer to amino acid therapy as Neuroadaptagen Amino Acid Therapy (,NAAT) a term used by Dr. Kenneth Blum, the key researcher in this type of therapy. We are going to explain why and how it works. As we mentioned before, some of this may be a bit hard to follow if you are unfamiliar with some of the scientific terms, but continue to stay with us. We want you to understand the science behind NAAT. We are sharing with you the most recent information available to us (at the time of this publishing) on how to attain dopamine homeostasis with NAAT therapy.

David: *I had maintained more than ten years of abstinence from alcohol when I first heard of amino acid therapy. While I had learned to cope with the discomfort of sobriety, I had found nothing that truly gave me relief. I still struggled with stimulus augmentation and stress sensitivity. Another addiction professional told me about an amino acid formulation and suggested I try it. I did, more because he asked me to than because I expected a positive result. I noticed the effect almost immediately. The major benefit was the reduction in stimulus augmentation. Everything seemed toned down. Life was less shrill. I felt less bombarded by sounds and things going on around me. In a word, I felt relief. It was as if I were wrapped in a soothing blanket. My internal molecules seemed to quiet and stop fighting me. I felt at ease. It felt as if I had taken a stone out of my shoe. The effect was so dramatic that Merlene noticed it right away. She said I seemed more relaxed and easy to be around. In fact, over time I discovered that any time I failed to take the amino acid supplement she would say, "Did you take your nutrients?" sometimes before even I realized that I had forgotten. I realize now that for the first time in my life I was functioning at a comfort level that seemed to begin in my brain, filtered throughout my body, and affected my behavior. Even though I still had some ups and downs with mood, this level of comfort became my normal state, and the ups and downs are much easier to deal with.*

The Brain and Amino Acids

Every living cell is produced in large part from amino acids. Reproducing, altering, or growing any type of cell requires a balance of the various amino acids. Human behavior—cognition, concentration, memory, mood, sleep, thirst, appetite, alertness, and emotions—involves functioning of the whole nervous system. The nervous system is regulated almost entirely by amino acids and their biochemical companions, vitamins and minerals.

As we mentioned earlier, neurotransmitters are produced from amino acids: Serotonin is produced from L-tryptophan; dopamine is produced from L-phenylalanine and L-tyrosine; endorphin and enkephalin levels are increased by D-phenylalanine; and glutamine is involved in the synthesis of GABA.

Amino acids and brain functioning go hand in hand. Neurotransmitters built from amino acids can fill their respective neuron receptors and nourish the brain with what you may be missing. Neurotransmitter balance—and imbalance—is related to amino acids. So, in a way, it is a no-brainer! The most important goal that should be embraced by addiction professionals and recovering people should be to restore neurotransmitters and neuroreceptors to their normal state and ensure "dopamine homeostasis." We can get there by upholding certain principles involving NAAT.[2]

While it has become obvious that we can nourish an impoverished brain with amino acids, it is not quite as easy as it sounds. This is because individual amino acids and their respective neurotransmitters do not work alone but form a novel and important network we call brain reward circuitry that, as we have already discussed, leads to the carefully modulated release of dopamine in the reward region of the brain. Although the process of how it works is quite complex, it is fairly easy to apply.

As we have already explained, drug craving and chronic abstinence symptoms are a result of malfunctions of the reward center of the brain involving certain neurotransmitters and the enzymes that control them. We now know that it is possible to reduce stress; reduce depression; increase glucose and neurotransmitter receptor sensitivity; and restore proper levels of key neurotransmitters with very selective amino acid supplementation. (Too many of the wrong amino acids will be counter productive and will reduce the benefit of the very carefully selective amino acids utilized in NAAT.

With NAAT, brain chemistry can be rebalanced resulting in rapid relief from cravings. Recovery is accelerated with relief from physical, mental, and emotional symptoms. In the short term, this therapy provides a jump start for recovery that allows people to better participate in the other aspects of treatment and to do so with more clarity and optimism. In the long term, it improves the quality and comfort of sobriety and reduces the risk of relapse.

If this sounds too good to be true or a dream for the future, let us assure you that it is already happening. It is not a gimmick. It isn't a theory. It has been researched and been found effective in the management of addiction recovery. It works.[3]

Essential and Nonessential Amino Acids

Amino acids are the building blocks of proteins, combining into tens of thousands of complex chains (called polypeptides) of differing links and complexities. (For example, human growth hormone is a chain of 191 amino acid molecules, while glutathione is a short chain of only three amino acids.) It is generally agreed that twenty amino acids (or twenty-one if you include L-taurine, which we do) are necessary for the creation of protein in the body. (Note: There are over 700 non-protein amino acids, which will not be discussed in this book.) Your body is able to produce many of these twenty-one amino acids from other amino acids already in the body.

Because the body normally manufactures them—and hence they do not have to be in foods we eat or supplements we take—these are called nonessential amino acids. It is important to keep in mind that nonessential does not mean these amino acids are unimportant. It simply means that, under ideal circumstances, it is not essential to consume food or supplements.

Forms of Amino Acids

Most amino acids, except glycine and taurine, can appear in two forms, the chemical structure of one being the mirror image of the other. These are called the D- form and the L- form. Products containing the L-form are by far more common in nature and more compatible with human biochemistry. All of the amino acids recommended in this book for the management of addiction are the L-form with one important exception: D-phenylalanine.[4]

The Brain Reward Cascade and Dopamine Homeostasis

The following select amino acids help produce the neurotransmitters most often involved in addiction and form the basis for NAAT: L-phenylalanine (increases dopamine), L-tryptophan and 5-hydroxy tryptophan (5-HTP) (increases serotonin), L-tyrosine (increases dopamine), L-glutamine (increases GABA), D-phenylalanine (increases endorphins). We should also point out that GABA is both an amino acid and a neurotransmitter.

These essential amino-acids are important because they are key building blocks for the brain neurotransmitters as detailed previously. Now we provide some information about these individual amino acids, especially as they relate to brain chemistry and the brain reward cascade.

L-TRYPTOPHAN

L-tryptophan increases the production of the neurotransmitter serotonin which may reduce cravings and help you relax and sleep. However, its main purpose is to stimulate serotonin receptors in the hypothalamus of the brain (part of the brain reward circuitry). By doing so, this action causes the release of the brain's endorphins.

D-PHENYLALANINE

One of the most important amino acids to bring about appropriate dopamine release and its homeostasis is D-phenylalanine. Its major action is to inhibit the enzyme that regulates the amount of endorphins in the brain.

In the 1970's Kenneth Blum began to explore the role of genetics on drug seeking behavior. He and his associates at the Institute of Behavorial Genetics at Colorado Unversity performed a number of experiments that helped to learn why some bred mice love alcohol and other strains do not. They found that loving alcohol or hating alcohol was due to the genetic trait of producing endogenous opioids (endorphins, enkephalins, etc.) in the brain. Specifically, mice that love alcohol have lower natural brain enkephalins than mice that hate alcohol. They found that when enkephalins were injected into the brains of the alcohol-loving mice, they stopped drinking alcohol. The next logical step was to find a way to increase the amount of enkephalins in the brain of alcohol loving mice. This was finally accomplished when D-phenylalanine was administered to these alcohol loving mice. Following 18 days of treatment, the scientists found that now the alcohol-loving mice stopped drinking alcohol and, in fact, looked like the mice that hated alcohol. When the brain was checked for enkephalins, there was no difference between alcohol-loving and alcohol-hating mice. This was the birth of amino-acid therapy for addiction!

L-GLUTAMINE

Glutamine produces GABA in the brain. However, it is important to know that, in providing the optimum amount of GABA, only small amounts of L-glutamine should be used in the amino acid regimen. This is so because of what we call the "GABA paradox." *If there is too much GABA activity, the amount of dopamine released into the synapse will be reduced way below normal.* This may cause "dopamine resistance" and could lead to a dopamine deficiency. On the other hand, if there is too little GABA activity and the amount of dopamine released is way above normal, schizophrenia can result. So we must be careful to provide the right amount of L-glutamine to enable the appropriate amount of dopamine to be released. (As we said above, you can take GABA, but it has trouble crossing the blood-brain barrier because it is already a neurotransmitter. So there is no way to know how much may actually reach the brain.) The GABA-dopamine relationship is more complex than we can explain here[5] and more complex than you can figure out on your own. For this reason it is best that you not try to apply amino acid therapy without the guidance or recommendations of someone who understands the science.

L-PHENYLALANINE

L-phenylalanine is an essential amino acid: that is, it must be obtained frequently from the diet in adequate quantities to meet the body's needs. Once in the brain, it can be converted into another amino acid, L-tyrosine, which in turn is used to synthesize (with the help of vitamin B6) the key neurotransmitter of reward—dopamine. It is known that only about 20% of L-Phenylalanine is converted to tyrosine and then to dopamine. Phenylalanine is available in three different forms: D-, L-, and DL-. (DL- is a combination of D- and L- and can be purchased as DLPA.) L-phenylalanine is the most common type (found in nature and in food) and is the form in which phenylalanine is incorporated into the body's proteins. Therefore, the most important purpose of this amino acid is conversion to tyrosine and subsequent conversion to dopamine.

L-Tyrosine

L-Tyrosine is very important because it is the only amino acid that directly regulates dopamine. Too little tyrosine means low dopamine; too much tyrosine means too much dopamine. In fact, cocaine causes damage to the brain because it affects the activity of tyrosine, and following cocaine abuse the levels of dopamine in the brain fall drastically and result in dopamine depletion. So we need L-tyrosine.

We do have some good news for carriers of the A1 form of the DRD2 gene (the gene form most often associated with reward deficiency syndrome). It has been found that they are able to convert tryosine to dopamine better than those that have the A2 form. This is because the activity of the enzyme that naturally converts tyrosine to dopamine is more sensitive in A1 carriers and yields higher dopamine levels. That is why foods that contain tyrosine may be beneficial. This trait may protect the A1 carrier despite having 30-40% fewer dopamine D2 receptors. A number of studies have shown that NAAT works better for carriers of the DRD2 A1 form than for the A2 carriers who need it less. That probably explains why A1 carriers have a much better rate of continuing NAAT than A2 carriers. They need it more and the results are more obvious. A1 carriers may never have gotten the needed amount of tyrosine, even at early age, putting them at greater risk for addiction. Since so many addicts are A1 carriers, this information should provide the impetus for supplementing with formulations that contain tyrosine, an important aspect often missed in treatment.

Other Important Ingredients Used in NAAT

In addition to amino acids there are other ingredients that have been found to be beneficial in the treatment of addiction.

Rhodiola Rosea

We know from genetic research that certain genes breakdown dopamine at various rates. Carriers of the fast-acting form of the COMT gene break down dopamine in the synapse four times faster than carriers of the slow acting form. We are reiterating this important fact to point out that by using an herbal called *rhodiola rosea* the fast acting gene can be blocked, and as such, this nutrient is able to convert a low dopamine state to dopamine homeostasis. In another example, one form of the mono-amine-oxidase (MAO) gene that causes a fast breakdown of dopamine in mitochondria can also be blocked by *rhodiola rosea*.[6]

Chromium Salts

The utilization of a known trace metal called chromium has been utilized as an alternative way of boosting serotonin in the brain. This occurs because chromium increases peripheral tryptophan to enter into the brain and therefore enhances the synthesis of serotonin. Interestingly, chromium also reduces blood sugar and increases the sensitivity of insulin at receptor sites. This effect has influence on brain dopamine function.[7]

Passion Flower

This is a very old herbal that has many effects in the brain. One of the most important effects is that it stimulates benzodiazepine receptors in place of GABA. This herbal may be helpful in stress reduction, but its use must be cautiously calculated so that it does not cause a GABA-like effect that could reduce required dopamine release. However, when it is used properly it has been shown to reduce cocaine and alcohol seeking behavior. The compelling question that remains is how to utilize this knowledge and apply its benefits to overcoming your addiction.

Considerations for Utilizing Neuroadaptagen Amino Acid Therapy (NAAT)

There are two commonly used approaches to attaining dopamine homeostasis: (1) targeting a specific neurotransmitter that may be deficient to increase production of that neurotransmitter[8] and (2) balancing the entire reward cascade with the appropriate amount of each ingredient to create the right ratio of serotonin, endorphins, GABA, and dopamine. By way of disclosure we want you to know that we support balancing the reward cascade. But while targeting a specific neurotransmitter has limitations, which we will point out, it has been used quite effectively for some time and is currently used in numerous treatment centers. So we mention it here because it served us well over many years when it was our only amino acid option for altering brain chemistry to aid recovery from addiction. And also because you may go to a treatment center or practitioner that uses this method. In that case you need to know that it has been found to be beneficial although more complicated to deliver and usually less effective.

TARGETING A SPECIFIC NEUROTRANSMITTER

There are two tasks in targeting a specific neurotransmitter: identifying which neurotransmitter is deficient and treating that deficiency by applying the amino acid and co-factors that will help the body produce more of that brain chemical. First you need to understand that short of a spinal tap or DNA test there is no definitive way to determine which neurotransmitter is low and that is not easily done. It is not done in treatment centers in America.[9] So when using this approach we take our best guess based on certain indicators. And sometimes we have to use trial and error to try to figure it out.

One method of identification that is commonly used is looking at symptoms. One group of symptoms may indicate low serotonin, another group might indicate an endorphin deficit. This is usually a pretty good place to start because symptoms often do reflect a specific deficiency. But quite often you will have symptoms from more than one group of symptoms. So should you take something to increase serotonin or something to increase endorphins? Or if you are depressed it may be due to a situational issue rather than low serotonin.

Some practitioners use a blood or urine test to identify a deficient neurotransmitter. If using this method you should be aware that these tests tell you what your neurotransmitter levels are at the *time of the test*. Neurotransmitter levels vary according to a number of factors such as when and what you ate and what activities you have been engaged in. There are many factors that alter brain chemistry.

Your drug of choice is an indicator of a specific deficiency. This works pretty well if you have a drug of choice. Some people don't. They use whatever is available to get high or they use drugs in combination. And different people use a drug for different reasons. Some people use alcohol to relax, others use it for stimulation, and others use it to escape.

Once identified, treating a deficiency is not just a matter of taking a certain amino acid. Amino acids need co-factors (other nutrients) to work effectively. You can buy amino acid formulations that already contain the appropriate co-factors. There are formulations that target serotonin, or endorphin, or GABA, or dopamine

A potential problem with applying a specific amino acid to enhance a specific neurotransmitter is that you can put the reward system further out of balance by increasing the level of one neurotransmitter. As an example, you will remember that too much GABA can result in too little dopamine. You may get an immediate calming effect from increasing GABA, but if in the long run you have less dopamine; you will be worse off. Remember that all roads lead to dopamine, and our goal is dopamine homeostasis.[10]

BALANCING THE REWARD CASCADE

There are now amino acid formulations that do not target a specific neurotransmitter but balance the entire reward circuitry of the brain. They provide the exact amount of different amino acids in the right proportion to produce the right amount of serotonin, endorphin, GABA, and dopamine for the optimal amount of dopamine to be released in the reward center of the brain creating dopamine homeostasis. To understand this better, it may help to look at how amino acid therapy has developed over the years.

After Dr. Blum had spent many years studying the neurochemistry of addiction, he began investigating ways to alter the brain chemistry of addicted people to give them the comfort needed to participate in the recovery process. After studying the genetics of addiction, Blum took the next logical step—correcting the neurotransmitter abnormalities with the natural substances that produce them, amino acids. He developed the first oral supplements of amino acids formulated specifically for people in recovery. At first he produced two formulations: one for people addicted to drugs that stimulate the nervous system and the other for people addicted to drugs that depress the nervous system.

These formulations worked to reduce cravings and chronic abstinence symptoms. But after many years of research, Blum realized that *it is not the action of any one neurotransmitter that matters but the interaction of all the neurotransmitters that work together to produce dopamine.* Now he has found that since alcohol, other drugs, food, and certain risky behaviors all share common neurochemical mechanisms, only one basic formula is needed to bring about dopamine homeostasis. He has now developed a formula that works by balancing the entire reward cascade rather than by targeting specific neurotransmitters. The proportion of each amino acid and herbal has been carefully calculated for optimum activity, and the current formula maximizes its dopamine promoting homeostatic state. Though dopamine has been identified as the primary neurotransmitter associated with addiction, it never works in isolation. It is the interaction of the various neurotransmitters that brings about a dopamine reward in the brain.

Something else to consider when choosing an amino acid product is that people absorb nutrients from the intestinal tract in different quantities and at different rates. One person might absorb 98% of the amino acids while another person may only absorb 8%. If you take an amino acid individually or in combination with other amino acids, there is no way to determine the appropriate dosage other than by trial and error. It is impossible to know how much of what goes into the mouth is actually absorbed into and utilized by the brain. The most recent formula is made with a technology that allows it to go directly into the blood stream and to the brain without going through the intestinal tract.

We rely on the research of Kenneth Blum because of the many studies that have been done to support his work and also because he has continued over many years to develop new and better formulations utilizing the most recent scientific knowledge. We encourage you to read the history of his research in the Appendix.

Merlene Miller, MA and David Miller, PhD

Guidelines for NAAT

In order to obtain the best results utilizing NAAT we encourage you to adhere to certain guidelines.

Take amino acid supplements on an empty stomach. To understand why, you need to know something about the blood brain barrier. Nutrients are carried throughout the body via the bloodstream. As these nutrients pass by, each organ reaches out and takes what it needs to maintain itself. Since there are substances in the bloodstream that can injure the brain, it has a highly selective, protective membrane that is difficult to penetrate. Certain proteins called transporter or carrier proteins move through the barrier and expedite the passage of select nutrients into the brain. If too many amino acids seek to cross into the brain at one time, the transporters become overloaded and only the amino acids in greatest supply are allowed in. If you take an amino acid supplement with a high-protein meal, the select amino acids found in the supplement may not be able to penetrate the blood brain barrier because other amino acids will compete with the needed ones and reduce the potency of the amino acid supplement. Taking the supplement on an empty stomach will eliminate that problem .

It is best not to take amino acids and herbals individually. We don't recommend that you try to figure out which neurotransmitter you are deficient in and target that neurotransmitter with specific amino acids. As we explained previously, unless there is rigorous objective evidence of specific neurotransmitter imbalance through genetic testing or cerebral spinal fluid analysis (not blood or urine), you cannot accurately pinpoint any actual deficit to target. In fact, the random targeting utilizing additional amino acids could lead to further neurotransmitter imbalance.

This is just a reminder that without consideration as to the appropriate ratio between nutrients, you may not get the result you are seeking. Certainly we are not suggesting that individual amino acids, along with other vitamins and minerals, will not help you. They will probably relieve some of the chronic abstinence symptoms you experience but not balance the entire reward cascade. It is best if you can take a supplement in which each amino acid and herbal has been carefully calculated for optimum activity maximizing its dopamine promoting homeostatic state.

Avoid adding nutrients that will ultimately block dopamine. The unwanted blocking of dopamine can occur through the enhancement of GABA by administering L-glutamine which helps synthesize GABA in the brain. Administering the substance GABA itself will, of course, block dopamine as it enters the brain. We must tell you that this information is not well known among clinicians and many clinicians incorrectly utilize this substance in large amounts. If you are in a facility that uses any type of amino acid therapy, ask that you not be given any supplement that enhances GABA to any significant extent. You may feel better at the time you take it, but in the long run, excessive GABA will deplete dopamine and you will feel worse.

Caution: Do not take L-phenylalanine if you are pregnant or nursing. Do not take it if you suffer from panic attacks or severe anxiety, both of which may be aggravated by adrenaline derived from L-phenylalanine. Do not take it if you suffer from skin cancer melanoma or phenylketonuria (PKU). Do not use it if you are taking monoamine oxidase (MAO) inhibitors. L-phenylalanine has been reported to cause hypertension in some people.

Why Food Is Not Enough

Since the primary source of amino acids is food, you may be asking if a deficiency can be resolved with diet alone. The answer is: maybe, but not likely. Certainly, foods are important and we will discuss that in another chapter. You can get L-tryptophan from milk to produce serotonin. You can eat meat, cheese, or eggs for tyrosine to produce dopamine. And these will help you. But diet alone is probably not enough to fix imbalances—for several reasons.

Modern farming, food processing, and cooking practices result in foods that may not provide the nutrition that our brains need. In addition, many people have food allergies and may not digest and absorb nutrients well. Add to that the fact that you may have a genetic condition, aggravated by addiction and stress, that has created a need for higher levels of amino acids than you can get from diet alone.

No Magic Bullet

We do not want to give you the impression that NAAT is a cure-all. There isn't one. While we are raving fans of NAAT, it is not a substitute for good nutrition or other aspects of healthful living. (That's why it's called supplementation, not substitution.) We strongly recommend that NAAT be used in conjunction with some of the other modalities we talk about in this book and that you participate in a support group. There is now good evidence that the program and traditions espoused by Alcoholics Anonymous or Narcotic Anonymous (NA) may be linked to known molecular neurobiology that impacts recovery.

We don't want you to believe that everyone who takes an amino acid supplement will get an immediate result. Some do if they need it. Sometimes it takes a while to get the full effect. And you may not always realize it is working because you are not going to get high. The purpose is to help you feel normal. It will help you get more reward from every-day activities so that you don't have to get high off drugs in order to feel good. Sometimes you don't realize how much it is helping you until you stop taking it and the old discomfort comes back.

Occasionally people do have mild side effects or an unusual reaction such as an upset stomach or headache especially with large doses of amino acids. In these instances no permanent harm will be done as the amino acids leave the body within one to four hours. Frequently the reaction occurs only in the first few days as the body adjusts. The benefits will probably prove to be well worth the persistence.

Experts do not agree on how long a recovering person needs to take an amino acid supplement. People with less severe addictions may be able to discontinue daily amino acid supplements after a relatively short period of time. But chronic relapsers, those with pre-existing reward deficiency conditions, and people who continue to be uncomfortable when abstinent need all the help they can get, probably for life (similar to what is seen with other chronic conditions such as diabetes). This means giving the brain—daily—what it cannot produce naturally. In this regard, Kenneth Blum and his associates have developed the first ever Genetic Addiction Risk Score (GARS). This one-time test can tell you if because of certain variant genes across the brain reward circuitry you have a genetic vulnerability to all addictive or reward deficiency behaviors.[11]

Although it is not everything you need for continuing sobriety, you will be surprised at how much better you will feel with NAAT. The good news is that NAAT is not a drug, having little to no side effects. It is a brain vitamin. You will not feel high. You will just feel more normal—happier and less irritable, more calm, rested and alert. In addition you will have noticeably fewer drug and carbohydrate cravings.

Merlene Miller, MA and David Miller, PhD

Why Aren't Prescription Medications the Solution?

Prescription drugs are not the answer to addiction because, in most cases, they do not treat the underlying problem. They often have side effects that become problems themselves or cause the person to stop taking them. A common problem is that many of the drugs used to treat addiction are addictive. There is no point in trading one addiction for another. And prescription drugs can pose a danger if people have a relapse of their primary addiction and have the medication in their system. Combining mood-altering substances can create a life-threatening synergistic effect in the body. And there may be unexpected reactions to some substances.

Some medications that are prescribed for addiction block the effects of certain addictive substances by blocking the pleasure centers of the brain. The idea here is that you won't drink or use drugs because you won't be able to experience the mood-altering effects. But these substances may also block the ability to get pleasure in other ways and lead to depression or thoughts of suicide. Before any prescription drugs are used, all natural methods should be tried. Every day you read of deaths because of prescription drugs. We know of no deaths due to any of the methods that we recommend.

The important message here is that, while they may have some utility, the continued use of many of FDA approved drugs that favor blocking dopamine (such as buprenorphin) may cause suicidal thoughts due to prolonged dopamine deficiency. This has already been observed with a dopamine-blocking drug called Acomplia which was used to treat obesity (and rejected by the FDA).

Scientific Evidence

Now with over 40 years of intense scientific exploration as detailed in the Appendix, NAAT has been extensively studied in pre-clinical and human trials. As reported in a detailed review article[12] on both animal and human models to date, NAAT variants have been shown to:

- enhance brain enkephalin levels in rodents;
- reduce alcohol-seeking behavior in mice;
- pharmacogenetically convert alcohol-preferring mice to non-preferring mice;
- reduce drug and alcohol withdrawal symptoms in humans, evidence of a lower BUD score (building up to drink), and no severe depression on the MMPI;
- reduce stress response for patients in addiction treatment as measured by the skin conductance level (SCL), and significantly improved Physical Scores and BESS Scores (behavioral, emotional, social and spiritual);
- decrease six-fold AMA (against medical advice) rates after detoxification when comparing NAAT variant to placebo;
- reduce craving for alcohol, heroin, cocaine, nicotine;
- reduce inappropriate sexual behavior;
- reduce post-traumatic stress (PTSD) symptoms such as lucid nightmares;
- in quantitative electroencephalic (qEEG) studies in humans, modulate theta power in anterior cingulate cortex (an area known for drug abuse relapse;
- activate the N. Accumbens as well as activate and improve the prefrontal-cerebellar-occipital neural network in abstinent heroin addicts with a single dose compared to placebo in a pilot study;
- show a significant Pearson correlation in terms of enhanced compliance to NAAT treatment by carriers with the DRD2 A1 allele relative to carriers of the normal compliment of DRD2 receptors in known obese patients;

- suggest the importance of low dopamine function in better treatment outcome;
- reduce BMI and loss of pounds using a customized DNA-based NAAT;
- reduce cocaine-induced dreams;
- increase libido;
- increase glucose receptor sensitivity;
- restore neurotransmitters such as endorphins, serotonin, GABA, and dopamine;
- significantly reduce stress, drug craving, depression, irritability, paranoia, anger, and anxiety in alcoholics;
- increase energy;
- increase self-confidence;
- increase six times the likelihood of completion of a twenty-eight-day treatment program with fewer incidents of relapse;
- lower by 50 percent drug hunger score in stimulant abusers as compared to control group;
- in outpatients over a one-year period reduce treatment drop-out rate to 4.6% compared to 37% for the control group with a relapse rate of 20 percent compared to 87%t for the control group;
- result in an average weight loss for carbohydrate abusers over a 90-day period with a relapse rate of 18% compared to loss of an average of ten pounds and an 82% relapse rate in the control group;
- show the following results in a study published in 1997: Two groups of dieters were monitored for two years after completing a medically monitored fast. During the fast, the dieters used a powdered nutritional drink (Optifast) in place of two or three meals each day. (It is now well recognized that liquid dieters can lose weight rapidly but soon regain it when they

go off the liquid diet. This is because the body has gone into starvation mode; when food is available again, the body stores it for future periods of starvation.) In this study, after completing the fast, one group took an amino acid formulation each day and the other group did not. At the end of two years, the amino acid group showed: a twofold decrease in percent overweight for both males and females; a 70% decrease in cravings for females and a 63% decrease in cravings for males; a 66% decrease in binge eating for females and a 41% decrease for males; only a 14.7% regain of weight lost while the control group regained 41.7% of their lost weight.

- increase compliance of narcotic antagonist treatment in former methadone users;
- using state of the art using Functional Magnetic Resonance (fMRI) increase resting state functional connectivity in abstinent heroin addicts.
- increase brain functional connectivity in the nucleus acumbns, hippocampus, hypothalamus, and cingyulate gyrus, all involved in craving and in drug reinstatement.
- increase connectivity volume in rodents showing that NAAT can enhance neuronal firing in the brain reward circuitry and may even lead to what has been called neuroplasticity for long-term effects. This takes on important meaning because NAAT has been shown to eliminate not only terrifying lucid nightmares but can convert these lucid dreams into happy ones. This is important for people having PTSD.

A Story of Recovery
Like so many others who find that the road to recovery turns out to be a mountain to climb, Brian was a chronic heroin relapser. He doesn't remember how many times he has been in

treatment—sometimes for a few days, a few times for months. One time he went in for detox and four hours later was calling his dealer. One time he stayed sober for two years. One time he stayed sober long enough to get married and have a baby. But when his wife discovered he was using heroin again, she took the baby and left. During his times of sobriety, he went to twelve-step meetings and talked about how grateful he was to be clean. He had an outgoing personality and everyone liked him. He seemed to enjoy life. But Brian had a secret. He never stopped thinking about using heroin. He told himself he only had to make it one day at a time. But every day was a little harder than the one before. He couldn't get rid of the thought that if he could just use heroin once his life would be better. He usually began using in secret and was able to keep anyone from knowing for quite a while. But eventually he would be caught; and back to treatment he would go. Clean again, but not happy, not comfortable. Everyone who had believed in him began to give up on him. He finally gave up on himself and decided there was no point in getting straight if he could never maintain it.

But Brian was fortunate. He had a friend who didn't give up on him. Joe kept encouraging Brian to try again. Joe heard about NAAT and told Brian about it. It was a hard sell, but Brian agreed to give it a try. What did he have to lose? He felt that his life was over anyway. And deep in his heart he yearned to be able to live a clean and sober life. He had a lot to live for.

As part of treatment Brian developed a plan for ongoing self care and a plan for changing his behavior if he began regressing toward relapse at any time. After just a few days Brian felt a sense of relief he had never experienced before. In fact, he felt even better than he had before he began using heroin. At first, Brian kept waiting for the other shoe to drop. He kept expecting the craving and the yearning for heroin to return, but it didn't. He went to outpatient treatment for some time, and it was different from how it had been in the past. He was able to think more clearly and better able to apply what he was learning to his life.

Brian cautiously began to rebuild his life. Even though he had been able to play the role of a happy sober person in the past, this time the difference was noticeable. There was something in Brian's appearance and demeanor that was new and different. He was, for the first time, comfortable without drugs. He still took life one day at a time, but instead of every day being harder than the one before, now every day was better.

He wasn't able to save his marriage, but he was able to become an active parent. In his distant past he had been an artist and began to paint again. He has been clean longer than ever before. But the length of sobriety isn't as important to Brian as the quality of life. He feels he is really living now, not just holding on.

Thanks to Dr..Kenneth Blum for his extensive contributions to this chapter. For information on NAAT products now available contact **NuPathways at 800-614-7714.** Ask for your *Staying Clean and Sober* discount.

Six

This Is Your Brain on Food

To this point we have discussed supplements that will improve the quality of sobriety and help prevent relapse. But supplements are not more important than the food you eat daily. Nutrition is one of the most important aspects of recovery. And the more we learn about the relationship of the brain to addiction and of nutrition to the functioning of the brain, the more we know that poor nutrition and problems in sobriety are very much related. In order to protect sobriety, you need a nutrition plan based on sound nutritional principles.

Whatever you do to get sober and whatever else you do to stay sober, good nutrition should be a central part of recovery. Good nutrition includes food as well as supplements. Longterm recovery from addiction requires healthful eating and an adequate supply of amino acids, vitamins, and minerals. Not for a short period of time; not just until you are feeling better; not just until the initial withdrawal and craving are gone. A person seeking freedom from the discomfort of addiction must make the same kind of commitment to healthful eating that a diabetic must make. We have no magic bullet to fix either the pancreas or the brain once and for all. Dysfunction of both requires special care on a regular basis.

However, we have to admit that good nutrition is a moving target. Just about the time we think we have it all figured out, along comes a new study that lets us know that nobody has all the answers. And then we have to find out if the new study is valid. Not all studies can be trusted completely. There is often more—or less—to the picture than we are told. Especially if the studies have been supported by an interest group that has something to gain or lose by the outcome of the study or report. And remember that you have to consider your own situation and weigh the information accordingly. For instance, it has been reported that one glass a wine a day may be good for your heart. But this is certainly not the case if you are a recovering alcoholic. One glass of wine a day may lead to several and finally a full blown relapse—certainly not good for your heart.

So do not take the information you get here, or anywhere else for that matter, as the last word on your health. Keep an open mind and learn as much as possible about nutrition. In this chapter we are not going to talk specifically about a diet to prevent cancer, to strengthen your heart, or to help you lose weight. You will need to take these things into consideration as you make a nutrition plan for yourself. And there is plenty of information out there. We will mainly talk about nutrition for your brain because there is not a lot of information available about that. A nutrition plan should be individualized for you by you. Only you know your particular needs and what will help you stick with your plan.

One of the first things to consider is that a good nutrition plan should be enjoyable to maintain. Eating is an important part of life that is associated with pleasure. When we think of a diet as something that restricts us and deprives us, we are not likely to keep doing it. As we talk about what is good for you in recovery, you need to think about not only how your nutrition can support recovery but also how enjoyable it will be.

Why Nutrition is So Important in Recovery

Food is the fuel the brain uses to function. And when your brain is not functioning properly you will feel unwell, unhappy, or anxious. Your stress levels will rise and stimulus augmentation will be heightened. You will not be able to think clearly and you will probably not sleep well. You will begin craving something to fill up the emptiness. If you want to feel good and enjoy life, you need to adequately feed your brain.

Proper nutrition is essential for a happy and healthy brain. We need protein, carbohydrates, and fat to provide energy, maintain the body, and feed the brain. Vitamins enable the body to properly utilize the protein, carbohydrates, and fat. Minerals (in addition to building bones and teeth, carrying oxygen to body cells, and maintaining muscle) help vitamins work efficiently. Water performs many functions and is essential to the survival of all cells. Fiber performs a useful role in digestion and provides a feeling of satisfaction.

Foods and Mood

In considering how food builds and maintains the body, let's not forget its very vital role in altering and maintaining mood. Depending on what amino acids they contain, some foods increase mental alertness, concentration, and energy while others are natural tranquilizers that calm feelings of anxiety and stress. But foods that calm you can also cause you to feel drowsy and mentally sluggish. What you eat and when you eat it can play an important part in your mood. Let's face it: *We self-regulate our mood continually with food.* Most of the time, we really don't know what we are doing and go for the quick fix rather than long-term well being. To maintain sobriety and feel good it is imperative that you be familiar with the various types of foods and the nutrition they supply.

FOODS FOR ALERTNESS
As you already know, the neurotransmitter tyrosine increases energy and alertness. Foods highest in tyrosine are foods derived from animal protein: chicken, turkey, pork, beef, dairy, and eggs. Moderate amounts of tyrosine are found in plant foods such as beans, corn, spinach, oatmeal, nuts, and seeds.

FOODS FOR RELAXATION
The neurotransmitter tryptophan, synthesized to serotonin, promotes relaxation and sleep. Foods high in tryptophan include turkey, green leafy vegetables, dairy products, bananas, pineapple, avocado, lentils, sesame seeds, and pumpkin. There are not many foods that contain tryptophan and those that do may not contain amounts sufficient to make it past the blood brain barrier if they are competing with other amino acids, especially tyrosine. However, carbohydrates helps carry the tryptophan to the brain. But if you eat a carbohydrate rich meal early in the day it can cause drowsiness. It is better to eat tryptophan rich foods and carbohydrates in the evening when you want to relax and prepare for sleep rather than for breakfast when you want to become alert and energized. A good bedtime snack is milk and toast. The bread will help the tryptophan in the milk reach your brain and help you sleep.

Protein, Protein, Protein

A very important thing to know about a diet for recovery is that *protein contains all of the essential amino acids.* Therefore, a high protein diet will give your brain more of the amino acids essential for its health. Think protein, protein, protein. Complete protein foods include meat, poultry, fish, eggs, and dairy products.

Protein not only feeds your brain and gives you energy, it also provides the body with the material it needs to replace worn tissue, fight infection, manufacture hormones and enzymes, and digest food. The body is damaged by heavy use of alcohol and other drugs and needs protein for rebuilding. The body stores very little protein, so you should eat it at least three times a day. And for enough energy—and your brain's sake—we recommend three meals and three snacks daily. You will probably feel best if your diet contains around 30 percent protein. And remember that most protein foods are rich in tyrosine.

HIGH-PROTEIN CAUTIONS

Keep in mind that high-protein diets do require some cautions. Before you go on a high-protein diet, get a physical examination to make sure your kidneys are healthy and functioning well. Do not go on a high-protein diet if you have any kind of kidney problem. The kidneys are forced to work harder when they have to process protein as opposed to carbohydrates. Diets that contain significant amounts of red meat, especially fried may increase the risk of cancer. So, here are some words of advice about eating red meat: Cook meat slowly with lower heat. Try baking or crock pot meals such as stews. High heat causes carcinogens to form. Broil rather than grill. Avoid nitrite-cured meats. Most cured cold cuts and meats such as hot dogs, bacon, and ham—contain nitrites that can spur formation of carcinogenic nitrosamines.

Red meat is usually high in fat—the bad saturated fat. A diet high in harmful fat poses many risks including that of heart disease. A high protein diet that is high in harmful fat is not a good idea regardless of the benefit to your brain chemistry.

LOW-FAT PROTEIN FOODS

But there are other good sources of animal protein that are low in fat or that contain good fat. Poultry and fish are, of course, the well known ones. Fish is one of the most important ingredients in your diet which we will discuss at more length later. But most of us get tired of a steady diet of chicken and fish. Try some alternatives.

Buffalo meat is red meat that is lower in fat than chicken but very tasty. If you have a hard time finding buffalo meat, get a group together and ask your grocer to stock it. Wild game also is usually low in fat and high in amino acids, so give it a try. Here's a great recipe for chili made with buffalo meat that you may want to try.

DAVE'S BUFFALO CHILI

2 lbs. ground buffalo
1 30-1/2 oz. can chili beans
1 28-oz. can diced tomatoes
1 pkg. Williams' Chilli Seasoning*
1 Tbsp. B-V concentrate
1 large onion
1 can V-8 juice
Brown bison in skillet. Place in crock pot with other ingredients. Slow cook for 6-8 hours.
*no salt, msg, or preservatives added

Other sources of low-fat or good-fat protein high in tyrosine are eggs, yogurt, feta cheese, and cottage cheese. Be creative and find ways to enjoy low-fat high tyrosine foods to increase your energy and your ability to concentrate.

Fats

Don't be afraid of fat. Fat provides the most concentrated source of energy, supplies essential fatty acids, and enables the body to absorb certain vitamins. Like carbohydrates, there are good fats and bad fats. Without enough of the right types of fats, the brain is deprived of critical nutrients and the possibility of depression and other mental disorders increases. The goal is not to lower your fat consumption but to lower your bad fat consumption. Our bodies need fat, and if we do not consume enough fat to give the body the energy it needs, we will crave simple carbs for fuel. An excellent way to relieve cravings for carbohydrates is to eat plenty of good fat. It is essential to your health and important to your recovery to learn which fats are good and which are bad for you.

Fats can be: saturated, monounsaturated, or polyunsaturated. These designations refer to the types of bonds that hold their carbon atom chains together. Trans-fatty acids, another type of fat, are created through hydrogenation.

Saturated fatty acids are primarily found in red meat and dairy products. You should eat most saturated fatty acids sparingly because the liver manufactures cholesterol, especially LDLs (the bad cholesterol) from them. You do not, however, want to eliminate them entirely from your diet, because they constitute at least 50 percent of cell membranes, giving them firmness and integrity. Saturated fatty acids play a vital role in maintaining healthy bones.[1] They lower Lp(a), a substance in the blood associated with heart disease.[2] Saturated fatty acids are needed by the body to utilize essential fatty acids.[3] The fat around the heart muscle is mostly saturated fat, and the heart draws on this reserve of fat in times of stress.[4] Eggs are a good source of saturated fat. Another good source is virgin coconut oil, which we will discuss shortly.

Monounsaturated fat is good fat. Olive oil and canola oil contain high amounts of monounsaturated fatty acids, 80 and 70 percent, respectively. The high consumption of olive oil in Mediterranean countries is considered to be one of the reasons why these countries have lower rates of heart disease.

Monounsaturated fat is believed to lower cholesterol and may assist in reducing heart disease. It provides essential fatty acids for healthy skin and the development of cells. Monounsaturated fat is also believed to offer protection against certain cancers such as breast and colon cancer.

Monounsaturated fats are typically high in vitamin E, an antioxidant vitamin that is usually in short supply in many Western diets. Cold-pressed extra-virgin olive oil, if not overheated, provides a range of phytochemicals and phenols that help to boost immunity and maintain good health. In addition to olive oil and canola oil, avocados, flaxseed, and most nuts also have high amounts of monounsaturated fat.

Polyunsaturated fatty acids have two or more double bonds. Oils that contain a high percentage of polyunsaturated fatty acids come from the following: corn, safflower, sunflower, peanut, cottonseed, soybean, fish, walnut, and flaxseed. Flaxseed oil and fish oil are the most highly unsaturated of all oils.

Fatty acids are the building blocks of fat. Essential fatty acids are necessary for human growth and cannot be manufactured in the body so we must get them from our diet. There are two families of essential fatty acids: omega-6 fatty acids and omega-3 fatty acids.

Most Americans consume adequate amounts of omega-6 fatty acids. The ratio of omega-6 to omega-3 fatty acids in your diet should be about

4:1. The typical Western diet contains approximately fourteen to twenty times more omega-6 fatty acids than omega-3s. Omega-6 fatty acids are most abundant in refined vegetable oils and red meat. Omega-3 fatty acids are found in foods such as fish, flaxseed oil, olive oil, and krill oil.

Omega-3 Oil Increases Size or Volume of Brain Structures Associated with Mood

People who have lower blood levels of omega-3 fatty acids are more likely to have a negative outlook and be more impulsive. Conversely, people with higher blood levels of omega-3 fatty acids were found to be more agreeable and less likely to report mild or moderate symptoms of depression.

Human participants who had high levels of long-chain omega-3 fatty acid intake had higher volumes of gray matter in areas of the brain associated with emotional arousal and regulation. These are the same areas where gray matter is reduced in people who have mood disorders such as major depressive disorder.

Sarah M. Conklin[5]

FISH OIL

Omega-3 fatty acids are found primarily in oily fish such as salmon, sardines, halibut, and mackerel. Fish-oil deficiency has been closely linked to addiction and co-existing conditions such as depression, anxiety, ADHD, cognitive impairment, and sleep disorders. You can consume an adequate amount of omega-3 fatty acids by eating three servings of fish a week. Of course, the benefits of fish will be counteracted if you fry fish in harmful fat or even good fat that changes its form when heated. Broil or bake your fish or fry it in palm oil or coconut oil (which will be discussed below). If you don't eat fish three times a week, be sure to take fish oil supplements.

KRILL OIL

In a perfect world, you would be able to get all the omega-3s you need by eating fish. But perhaps you do not like fish. Or perhaps you are rightfully concerned about studies that show that eating fish can potentially expose you to a high degree of contamination with industrial pollutants and toxins, such as mercury, PCBs, heavy metals, and radioactive poisons.

Fortunately, you can get the same benefits from krill oil. Krill are shrimp-like marine invertebrates. While fish oil is very perishable, krill oil is very stable because it contains potent antioxidants that protect the oil. It has been claimed that krill oil is perhaps one of the best brain-building foods available. Krill oil improves concentration, memory, learning, and mood. In addition to being a good brain food, krill oil is good for your heart, joints, cell membranes, liver, immune system, and skin.

EXTRA-VIRGIN OLIVE OIL

The greatest exponent of monounsaturated fat is olive oil. Olive oil is a natural juice, the only vegetable oil that can be consumed as it comes from the fruit. The beneficial health effects of olive oil are due to both its high content of monounsaturated fatty acids and its high content of antioxidants.

Olive oil is very well tolerated by the stomach. In fact, olive oil's protective function has a beneficial effect on ulcers and gastritis.

Generally, olive oil is extracted by pressing or crushing olives. Olive oil comes in different varieties, depending on the amount of processing involved. Varieties include:

- Extra virgin: considered the best, least processed, comprising the oil from the first pressing of the olives
- Virgin: from the second pressing.
- Pure: undergoes some processing, such as filtering and refining.
- Light: undergoes considerable processing and only retains a very mild olive flavor.

When buying olive oil, look for a high-quality extra-virgin oil. The less the olive oil is handled, the closer to its natural state, the better the oil. Keep olive oil in a cool and dark place, tightly sealed. Oxygen promotes rancidity. Do not buy into the hype that canola oil is superior to olive oil due to its concentration of monounsaturated fatty acids. Olive oil is far superior and has been around for thousands of years. If the taste of olive oil is a problem, or if you are frying or sautéing food, then you should consider coconut oil.

Virgin Coconut Oil[6]

We have very good news about coconut oil. It is good for you. That is, virgin coconut oil—or extra-virgin coconut oil. (Virgin and extra-virgin coconut oil are the same thing. Some manufacturers or retailers refer to virgin coconut oil as extra virgin. There is no difference in processing as there is with virgin and extra-virgin olive oil.) There is a difference, however, between virgin coconut oil and RBD coconut oil. RBD stands for refined, bleached, and deodorized. It is made from copra, the dried meat of the coconut. Virgin coconut oil, which is made from fresh coconut meat, is visibly clear and retains the scent and taste of coconuts.

Many nutritionally misinformed people consider use of coconut oil unwise due its nearly exclusive content of saturated fat. To understand why this is not true it is necessary to understand the chemical structure or the length of fatty acid chains.

Merlene Miller, MA and David Miller, PhD

Coconut oil is comprised of medium-chain fatty acids (MCFAs). Coconut oil is nature's richest source of these healthy fatty acids. Most vegetable or seed oils are composed of long-chain fatty acids. LCFAs are difficult for the body to break down, and they put more strain on the pancreas, the liver, and the digestive system. LCFAs are predominantly stored in the body as fat.

The MCFAs in coconut oil are healthier than LCFAs because they are smaller, so they permeate cell membranes easily. They are easily digested and are sent directly to your liver where they are immediately converted into energy rather than being stored as fat. Due to its stability and resistance to oxidation and free-radical formation, you can store coconut oil at room temperature for two years or more and it will not become rancid. However, don't store it in direct sunlight.

In the 1930s, Dr. Weston Price, a dentist, traveled throughout the South Pacific examining traditional diets and their effect on dental and overall health. He found that those who ate diets high in coconut products were healthy and trim, despite the high fat concentration in their diet.

Similarly, in 1981, researchers studied populations on two Polynesian atolls. Coconut was the chief source of caloric energy in both groups. The results, published in the *American Journal of Clinical Nutrition*, demonstrated that both populations exhibited positive vascular health. There was no evidence that the high saturated fat intake had a harmful effect in these populations.

Extra-virgin olive oil is healthier than coconut oil if it is not heated. It is an omega-3 fat and works great as a salad dressing. However, it is not the best oil to cook with. Due to its chemical structure, cooking makes it susceptible to oxidative damage. And polyunsaturated fats—which include common vegetable oils such as corn, soy, safflower, sunflower, and canola—are the worst oils to use in cooking. This is because their double bonds are highly susceptible to heat damage.

Frying destroys the antioxidants in these oils and oxidizes the oils, which causes far more damage.

Coconut oil is the only oil that is stable enough to resist heat-induced damage, so you can use coconut oil instead of butter, olive oil, vegetable oil, or any other type of oil called for in recipes. Coconut oil is very stable even at high temperatures. However, it is best not to heat it beyond its smoke point as this will deteriorate the oil and turn it yellow. (If coconut oil has turned dark yellow it should be discarded.) The smoke point of coconut oil can be increased by combining it with virgin palm oil. Both of these oils have a much higher smoke point and are suitable for high heat, even for deep frying.

You have probably heard that breast milk is packed with nutrients and disease-fighting ingredients that help keep babies healthy. Coconut oil contains one of the same compounds, lauric acid, that helps strengthen the immune system. Lauric acid is the predominant type of MCFA in coconut oil. In fact, a volume of research has been done establishing the ability of lauric acid to enhance immunity. Outside of mother's milk, coconut oil is nature's most plentiful source of lauric acid.

The numerous health benefits of coconut oil are finally reaching the mainstream. Benefits include promoting heart health, promoting proper weight maintenance, supporting the immune system, improving metabolism, providing an immediate energy source, keeping skin healthy, and supporting healthy thyroid function. To get full health benefits of coconut oil, try to consume three to four tablespoons per day.

Just a word or two of caution: Be sure to purchase virgin coconut oil that has not been refined, has no chemicals added, has no hydrogenation, and is made without heat processing. And don't pay any attention to some ads that claim that their coconut oil is better because it is more raw and therefore contains more enzymes. If coconut oil contained enzymes it would quickly deteriorate and would not have some of the benefits we have been telling you about. Also we want to be sure you don't think that you are getting omega-3 fatty acids in coconut oil. There are none. You still need to get those from fish, fish oil, and other foods high in omega-3.

In our home, coconut oil is a mainstay. It is the only oil we use, (except for olive oil on salads). It enables us to enjoy fried food, which we considered off limits before we discovered the health benefits of coconut oil. And remember what we said earlier: You are more apt to stick with healthy eating if you enjoy it. With coconut oil you can fry, stir-fry, or sauté. You can make your own mayonnaise. And for a dose of lauric acid, you can put some into a smoothie or other healthy snack. So enjoy. No cholesterol. No trans-fats. No guilt. No downside.

AVOID TRANS-FATTY ACIDS

Trans-fatty acids behave in many ways like saturated fat, including raising your LDL (bad) cholesterol. They are formed through a process of heating vegetable oil into solids like margarine and shortening (hydrogenating). They are often added to processed foods, allowing them to be shipped in warm, humid weather and left on grocery store shelves for months. Look for the words *hydrogenated* or *partially hydrogenated* in the list of ingredients to see if trans-fat is included. Trans-fatty acids push both blood cholesterol levels (LDL and HDL) in the wrong direction. They also interfere with essential-fatty-acid metabolism.

Foods high in trans-fatty acids include: biscuit mixes and dough, cakes and cake mixes, cinnamon rolls, cookies and cookie mixes, corn chips, crackers, doughnuts, granola, frozen desserts (not ice cream), muffin mixes, pastries in general, pie crusts and pie crust mixes, popcorn (flavored), potato chips, shortening, tortillas, and tortilla chips. The good news is that more of these foods are now being produced without transfatty acids. Be sure to read the labels so you'll know what you are buying.

Carbohydrates

Carbohydrates are a major energy source and help us use other nutrients. Carbohydrates also help produce serotonin. The lowcarb craze may have you thinking that carbs are bad for you. Like fat, however, there are good carbs and bad carbs. And you need the good carbs—for energy and for serotonin production.

When the body digests food, it converts carbohydrates to a type of sugar called glucose. As the level of glucose rises in the bloodstream, the pancreas releases insulin which helps move the glucose into the body's many cells. Once glucose enters the cells it is either burned for energy or converted to and stored as fat.

There are two types of carbohydrates: simple and complex. The big difference is in how quickly the body processes them into glucose. Simple carbs are processed quickly, while complex carbs are processed more slowly. The rate at which foods are processed into glucose is sometimes referred to as the glycemic load. Simple carbs are primarily sweets and white flour foods, and complex carbs are whole grains, legumes, and some vegetables and nuts.

The problem with simple carbs is that they give you a surge of energy that is soon followed by a letdown. This occurs because the pancreas releases insulin to compensate for the rush of sugar. The body then releases adrenaline to remove the insulin, which in turn produces that letdown feeling, which triggers a desire for more sweets to raise your blood sugar level for another surge of energy. If your blood sugar is low, you may feel moody, fatigued, confused, anxious, and irritable. All your chronic abstinence symptoms are intensified. Simple carbohydrates, then, contribute to mood swings, low energy, and cravings.

Complex carbohydrates are also made up of sugars, but the sugar molecules are strung together to form longer, more complex chains, so they're absorbed more gradually into the bloodstream. As a result, your brain does not get the sudden surge of sugar that it gets from simple carbs. Complex carbohydrates provide energy without the surge and without the letdown. They also give you a wider array of vitamins and minerals that your body cannot get from a strict high protein diet. A complex carbohydrate snack in the evening with some milk will provide tryptophan to increase serotonin to help you relax and sleep.

While we've presented a lot of information about nutrition, remember that the most important thing is to be moderate and sensible. Try to replace bad fats with good fats, bad carbs with good carbs. If you eat simple carbs once in a while, try to eat them with high fiber or good-fat foods. (Fiber and fat slow the rate at which carbohydrates are absorbed into the bloodstream.) And eat them late in the day when you want to relax rather than when you want to be alert.

In addition to selecting whole grains instead of processed grains and restricting white foods, here are some other ways you can get the serotonin and nutritional benefits of carbohydrates while lowering your glycemic load.

- Eat more legumes (dried beans, lentils and nuts).
- Eat more high-fiber fruits and vegetables.
- Add vinegar or lemon juice to carbs; the acid lowers the glycemic load as much as 30 percent. Eat a green salad with acidic dressing along with carbohydrate foods.
- Choose old-fashioned or steel-ground oatmeal over highly processed cereals.
- Eat brown rice and basmati rice, as well as wild rice (not actually rice but high in fiber, has a low glycemic load, and tastes very good).
- Eat a bit of protein or good fat along with carbohydrates.

The Story of the Potato

The potato is a paradoxical food. For a while, we were told that potatoes were high in starch (sugar) and should be eaten sparingly. At one time, First Lady Rosalynn Carter announced that her family was going to start eating better and cut out potatoes. But the potato industry responded by telling us it is not the potato, but what we put on it that is bad, and that potatoes are high in many of the vitamins and minerals we need. Good for us without the bad toppings. So some of us learned to enjoy our potatoes plain, leaving off the butter and sour cream. Recently, we have been hit with some bad news again. It is the potato. Researchers are telling us that eating a baked potato is the same as eating a half cup of sugar. Oh, wow! But they aren't telling us the whole story. That is true only if you eat it plain, on an empty stomach, with nothing on it or with it. Butter or sour cream slows the absorption process so it goes into the blood stream more slowly. If you substitute a good fat for butter or use low-fat sour cream, you can get the many nutrients in potatoes without spiking your blood sugar.

SUGAR AND OTHER SWEETENERS

We have been pointing out that simple carbohydrates are not the best choice for your diet. However, most people enjoy something sweet at least occasionally. If you eat sugar once in a while, do it in moderation. Avoid concentrated sweets such as sugared soft drinks, pies, cake icing, and candy. You can also eat things that are sweetened with substances other than processed sugar. But there are some things you need to consider when you do. Honey and molasses are simple carbohydrates and cause the same reaction in your brain as refined sugar. Honey does have trace amounts of vitamins not found in processed sugar and it is also an antioxidant. But it is still a simple carb and will have the same effect on your blood sugar and mood as other simple carbs.

Many people replace sugar with artificial sweeteners, but there is some controversy as to whether or not some artificial sweeteners are safe. Most are better for you than sugar and some of the reports and messages about them have been promoted by the sugar industry. Don't believe everything you hear, but it doesn't hurt to be cautious.

Processed fructose is a good choice if you aren't worried about the calories. It does not require insulin to make it available for energy in the body so it does not affect blood sugar levels. Fructose adds the same number of calories as sugar, however, so you don't hear much about it as most people want to avoid excess calories. (Don't take this to mean that all fruit is sweetened with fructose and therefore doesn't affect blood sugar. Different fruits have different sugars. Grapes are primarily sucrose.)

Complementary Protein

Although it is important to consume the full range of amino acids, it is not necessary to get them all from meat, fish, poultry, and other complete protein foods. In fact, because of their high fat content—as well as the use of antibiotics and other chemicals in the raising of poultry and cattle—most of those foods should be eaten in moderation only. Complete protein contains all the essential amino acids. Complex carbohydrates (incomplete protein) contain some of them. You can combine partial protein foods to make complete protein.

These are grains, legumes, and some leafy green vegetables. Brown rice and beans each lacks one or more of the necessary amino acids for complete protein. But when you combine the two, or when you combine either one with any number of other complex carbohydrate foods, you form a complete protein that is a high-quality substitute for meat. To make a complete protein, combine beans with brown rice, corn, nuts, seeds, or wheat.

As a matter of fact, combinations of legumes (such as beans, peanuts, peas) with almost any grains, nuts, or seeds will make a complete protein. In addition, cornmeal fortified with the amino acid L-lysine makes a complete protein. A meal of beans and corn bread provides complete protein without meat.

Another good way of adding protein to meals is to add nuts and seeds to salads and vegetable casseroles. Add protein-rich snacks as often as possible. Eat whole-grain bread with nut butters or a handful of nuts and seeds.

Remember, plant protein does not provide as much tyrosine as animal sources. If you choose to get your protein by reducing meat intake and consuming more combined carbohydrates, you may want to also add a little cottage cheese, skim milk, or eggs if you need the tyrosine.

Vitamins and Minerals

Vitamins enable the body to use the protein, carbohydrates, and fat for fuel and maintenance. We need a variety of foods, particularly fruits and vegetables, to get all the essential vitamins. You should eat five to eight servings of fruits and vegetables a day. Vitamin B12 (without which we develop pernicious anemia) is available only in animal foods. If you are a vegetarian, make sure you take a vitamin B12 supplement. Take it as a sublingual for maximum utilization by the body.

Minerals are necessary for building healthy bones and teeth, for carrying oxygen to body cells, and for maintaining muscle tone. They also help vitamins work efficiently. Calcium, necessary for building and maintaining bones and teeth, is found primarily in dairy products. Because dairy foods are characteristically high in fat, you should take special care to get adequate calcium if you reduce your fat intake. You can eat low-fat dairy products such as yogurt and low-fat cheeses, or get calcium from green leafy vegetables such as broccoli and collard greens.

Fiber

Fiber has no nutritive value, but it performs a useful role in digestion. Fiber contributes to good health and provides a feeling of satisfaction when we eat. It increases the feeling of satiation and reduces hunger and craving. High-fiber foods require more chewing, which helps us to eat more slowly, and slow eaters usually feel more satisfied. High-fiber foods include whole grains, fruits and vegetables, and seeds.

When to Eat

Very simply, you need to eat tyrosine rich foods when you want to be alert and tryptophan rich foods when you want to relax. To avoid hunger, eat several times during the day. How often you eat can vary, but it is important not to get hungry. We should eat smaller amounts more often to avoid getting hungry and eating the wrong foods. In recovery one of the major things we are trying to accomplish is to avoid cravings. Hunger creates cravings. And when you are really hungry, you will eat whatever is fastest, not what is best for you.

A nutritious breakfast provides the initial energy we need; it sets us up to function well throughout the day. Sara used to go all day without eating, thinking she was cutting calories. But by dinner time she would grab the fastest and easiest foods she could find, because she was too hungry to take time to cook. Usually the most convenient foods are not the most nutritious or the most satisfying. Once she started eating, she found it difficult to stop. She ended up eating more than if she had eaten breakfast and lunch. Now that her self-care plan includes eating regular meals, she has more energy all day long. She now realizes she was depriving her body of the fuel it needed for her busy life.

Avoiding Trigger Foods

Trigger foods are those that, when eaten, cause you to want to eat more—and more. Sweets are the most common trigger food. Complex carbohydrates are less likely to trigger cravings and are much easier to eat in reasonable amounts. Balance, balance, balance is the watchword. Carbohydrate binges are less likely to occur if you balance your carbs with high protein rather than trying to eliminate them completely.

If you attend a meeting of Alcoholics Anonymous you may find lots of coffee, lots of cigarette smoke, and sometimes a platter of donuts. It has been found that when alcoholics stop drinking or other drug addicts give up their drug of choice, they increase their intake of sugar, caffeine, and nicotine. Why? Because they need something to satisfy the craving created by removing the drug upon which they were dependent.

While this is sometimes encouraged or at least justified with the statement that eating sweets is better than drinking, in the long run, it is not a good alternative. Yes, for an alcoholic, eating sweets is better than drinking. But the fact is, it does not reduce craving and may make it more difficult to stay sober. The cravings that continue to plague the abstinent addict are an indication that the underlying problem has not been addressed. The brain is still crying out for something it is not getting.

How does the brain get what it needs to eliminate craving and provide a sense of well-being? Remember, craving is a neurotransmitter problem; neurotransmitters are made from amino acids. So what is the brain crying out for? Right. Proper nutrition.

Sugar and caffeine do not work to relieve cravings. It only seems like it at the moment. Like other drugs, they provide temporary relief. But the relief is quickly replaced by intensified craving. So these new substances create the same cycle of relief and craving that the drug of choice previously provided. And alcoholics or heroin addicts soon find themselves addicted to the substitute. What works is feeding the brain what it needs for neurotransmitter replacement.

There is a wide variety of opinion about the extent to which we should avoid trigger foods. Some people say trigger foods are like alcohol for an alcoholic and should be eliminated entirely, but for most people that is unrealistic. For some of us, the sense of deprivation that comes from identifying forbidden foods— foods we can never eat—creates stronger cravings than eating the foods in moderation.

There is no simple answer to this. And there certainly is not one that applies to everyone. But it is important to recognize that nutrition is an important part of recovery and that certain foods can trigger cravings for foods that do not feed our brains. But if you believe that by permanently depriving yourself of certain foods you risk bingeing on them to relieve the pain of feeling deprived, include them in your nutrition plan in a controlled way. Some people allow a treat periodically as part of their nutrition plan to relieve feelings of unrelenting deprivation. To eat the treat in moderation, follow a control plan for managing the craving that is triggered.

Sue occasionally gets a small ice cream cone, away from home, and then takes a walk in the park. She takes a small bag of nuts (high in protein) with her to offset the sugar. When the ice cream is gone, more is not readily available, and the exercise helps to relieve the craving. For her, this is much better than eating a bowl of ice cream at home. Ice cream in the freezer continues to call to her until she goes and gets more—and more and more.

When you eat a high protein diet you will be surprised to find that cravings are greatly reduced, even for carbohydrates. If your tendency is to grab a cookie when you are uncomfortable and find yourself bingeing on sweets, try eating some protein or complex carbohydrates instead of the cookies. You will feel more satisfied and less tempted to go for the ice cream. You will have more energy and feel less anxious. Your brain is getting what it needs to produce the feel-good neurotransmitters that need to be replenished.

Caffeine

Caffeine stimulates the release of neurotransmitters that make you feel energized. In moderation caffeine will not hurt you. And there may be some benefits for you. But five or six cups of coffee or bottles of cola a day can cause high anxiety. And you can become addicted to caffeine. If you find yourself drinking more than two or three cups of coffee a day or gradually increasing the amount you drink, you should cut back. Sugared soft drinks have other harmful ingredients and should be avoided completely or at least drunk only in moderation.

Weight

Many chemically addicted people are either overweight or underweight due to poor eating habits. Proper eating habits will probably correct an underweight problem fairly rapidly. A problem with obesity is not usually as easily corrected. A person can be overweight and still suffer from malnutrition. A weight reduction program should be undertaken carefully, with the help and advice of a physician.

Immediate weight loss in early sobriety may not be wise because of the stress related to dieting. This, along with the stress of adjusting to sobriety and a new lifestyle, may be more than you are ready to cope with. Talk to your doctor. It may be wise to establish and practice a good nutritional program along with making the other lifestyle adjustments necessary for recovery before thinking of losing weight.

If you decide to lose weight, do so sensibly. Beware of rapid weight-loss diets. They can be harmful to your health and very stressful. Be satisfied with gradual loss. Continue to eat a balanced diet and avoid hunger. Increase your exercise as well as decreasing calories. It is the combination that makes for the most successful weight-loss plan. A focus on good health rather than attaining an unrealistic weight goal usually achieves the best results.

A Modified Mediterranean Diet

We understand that figuring out how to eat nutritiously can be complicated and inconvenient sometimes. So we are going to recommend an eating plan for you that can make your life simpler while you enjoy healthy eating. The closest diet to what we have been recommending is the Mediterranean Diet. You can modify it according to your own preferences and according to some of the suggestions we have already made.

The Mediterranean Diet is a way of eating that cultures throughout the Mediterranean have practiced for centuries. Scientific studies associate this type of diet with longer lives and less disease.

12 Steps for Nutritious Eating

1. Eat nutrient-dense foods: Limit intake of simple carbohydrates, avoid empty-calorie junk foods.
2. Learn to read labels: Avoid overly processed foods with artificial ingredients and preservatives.
3. Eat 5–8 servings of fresh fruits and vegetables daily.
4. Get plenty of omega-3 fatty acids: Eat 2–3 servings of oily fish weekly and consume nuts and seeds daily.
5. Consume a balance of good fats; avoid bad fats. Use only coconut oil for cooking.
6. Eat three small meals and three snacks daily, beginning each day with a nutritious, balanced breakfast.
7. Snack between meals on nuts, seeds, fresh fruits (especially berries), and dark chocolate.
8. Eat slowly and chew thoroughly.
9. Supplement daily with amino acids, vitamins, and minerals.
10. Drink purified water (reverse osmosis preferred).
11. Avoid fruit juices: Chew your foods; don't drink them.
12. Avoid soft drinks and minimize coffee consumption; drink green tea or black tea instead.

Thanks to Bridging the Gaps for contributing to this list.

This diet is characterized by the following:

- High intake of vegetables, fruits, legumes, nuts, and seeds; whole-grain cereals and pastas; healthy monounsaturated fats like olive oil.
- Moderate to high intake of wild-caught fish
- Moderate intake of eggs and poultry; low fat dairy products
- Low intake of red meat and saturated fatty acids from meats and dairy.

Good nutrition feeds the brain. A well-functioning brain is the key to long-term sobriety. While this is sometimes mentioned in conventional treatment and occasionally in AA, it is seldom emphasized. The role of nutrition cannot be overstated. Addiction is a disease of the brain. Recovery requires feeding the brain.

Seven

ACUPUNCTURE, AURICULOTHERAPY, AND CRANIAL ELECTRICAL STIMULATION

I n the last few years, acupuncture and auricular therapy have been used increasingly to treat substance abuse disorders. Though more research is needed, numerous studies have validated the use of these therapies. Since scientific research shows that addiction, withdrawal, and chronic abstinence symptoms are related to chemicals in the nervous system and to stress regulating hormones in the body, it is reasonable that all remedies that affect these systems be explored when seeking therapy that works in the treatment of addiction.

Acupuncture[1]
Acupuncture dates back thousands of years. Yet, in the United States it has only recently begun to be recognized as a valid form of treatment for a variety of health conditions. There is strong evidence that it works, especially in the alleviation of pain. It has been used successfully as anesthesia for animals—and placebos don't work with animals.

Merlene Miller, MA and David Miller, PhD

Traditionally, acupuncture healers seek to restore the balance of two complementary energy forces (yin and yang) that travel through the body by way of channels called meridians. These energy forces crisscross the arms, legs, trunk, and head and course deep within the tissues. These energy forces must be in balance for our vital life functions—including physical, emotional, mental, and spiritual states—to operate correctly. The meridians surface at various locations—called acupuncture points—on the body, each of which is associated with one or more specific organ. The idea is that the organs can be influenced by stimulating an appropriate acupuncture point.

Acupuncture involves stimulation of these points on the skin with ultra fine needles that are manipulated manually, and sometimes electrically. It is said that acupuncture moves energy. The ancient explanation for the effectiveness of acupuncture is that when conditions interfere with the energy flow through the meridians, toxins build up in the body and block body systems from functioning optimally. Stimulating acupuncture points releases the energy flow, and balance is restored.

Western scientists suggest a different or additional explanation for the effectiveness of acupuncture: mobilization of endorphins in the reward system of the brain. This theory is supported by the fact that experimental animals, when given naloxone (a chemical that blocks endorphins) do not respond to acupuncture. As we have stated previously, the endorphins reduce pain even more effectively than narcotics and without the side effects.

There is no tangible evidence of the existence of acupuncture meridians. They cannot be touched or dissected. However, under a microscope acupuncture points appear to have a greater concentration of nerve endings than other skin locations. And electric skin conductivity, which can be measured, is greater at these points.

Concerning the safety of acupuncture, there is always potential harm when a sharp instrument penetrates the body. However, professionals using sterilized needles will seldom do any harm. We advise that you make sure the needles used on you are disposable—the most sure method of preventing transmission of infections like HIV/AIDS and hepatitis. Most states require acupuncturists to pass a course on infection control and proper handling of equipment.

The FDA has approved the use of acupuncture needles as medical devices. Some states restrict the practice of acupuncture to licensed doctors; other states and Washington, DC, permit non-physicians who complete a training course and pass a certifying exam to use acupuncture.

Specialists in pain management often use acupuncture. If you are a recovering addict and are abstaining from mood-altering substances, such as painkillers, acupuncture may be a good alternative for pain relief. People who suffer from back pain, bursitis, osteoarthritis, and headaches can benefit from acupuncture. In a study in California, eleven women plagued by recurring menstrual cramps were treated with acupuncture once a week. The same number of women received painkillers. After three months, ten of the women in the acupuncture group had significant relief. The others reported no change.[2]

Acu-detox (Ear Acupuncture)[3]

About 2,500 years ago, it was discovered that there are points in the ear that, when manipulated with needles, are effective in relieving the discomfort of withdrawal from opium. In more recent times Hsaing Lai Weng successfully applied electrical stimulation to needles inserted in the ear to relieve opiate withdrawal symptoms. Over several years Michael Smith, a physician at Lincoln Hospital in Bronx, New York, and his associates refined the detox protocol into five ear points that are manipulated with needles. Currently his protocol is utilized in numerous settings including drug treatment programs, jails, prisons, and drug courts.

While acu-detox has been found to be very beneficial, keep in mind that it is limited to detoxification from opiate-type drugs such as heroin, methadone, barbiturates and alcohol but has not been found to be helpful in detox from stimulants such as cocaine. And it is a detoxification tool, not a tool for ongoing recovery.

Ear acupuncture is an ancient discipline that has stood the test of time. Even though there is not strong scientific research to show how and why it works, there is plenty of anecdotal evidence to demonstrate its worth. When ear acupuncture is used in an inpatient detoxification setting, the severity of withdrawal is reduced and seizures can be controlled. It is usually done twice a day in a group setting for forty-five to ninety minutes.

Needle-less Auricular Therapy (Auriculotherapy)[4]

Although the term *auriculotherapy* is sometimes used to refer to any type of ear therapy, including ear acupuncture, we use it here to describe a needle-less procedure that utilizes four cranial nerves and three cervical ganglia within the ear, not acupuncture points. Auriculotherapy uses a microcurrent device to diagnose and treat those nerves that are a direct entry to the brain and spinal cord. Auriculotherapy is used to identify the location and measurement of an abnormal nerve point and then to treat that point with micro-amp current at a specific frequency depending on where the point is located.

Dr. Paul Nogier laid the groundwork of auriculotherapy in the 1950s. He discovered that auricular nerves form a microsystem. A microsystem is a small location in the body that represents the whole body. As with other microsystems—foot (reflexology), eye (iridology), scalp, or hand (Su Jok)—there are areas in the ear that correspond to specific systems of the body.

Nogier first used cautery to intervene at locations of the ear, then needles, and finally milli-amp current, which was the most successful. Later, other researchers upgraded to micro-amp current, which has worked the best and is almost imperceptible to the patient. These microcurrents were successful in relieving pain and caused no trauma to the patients.

Auriculotherapy practitioners use a hand-held device first to locate abnormal points of increased skin conductivity on the ear and then to treat those identified points. The nervous system is tonal, meaning the nerves function at a specific frequency, measured in hertz (Hz). Hertz is defined as cycles per second, or how many times something occurs within a second—its frequency. The auricular nerves function at 5 Hz, 10 Hz, or 20 Hz.

Auriculotherapy points manifest as points of increased skin conductivity only if there is a problem in the corresponding part of the body which the ear point represents. Once the points have been located, the microcurrent device is used to stimulate the nerve to decrease skin conductivity at that location. The less conductive, the healthier it is until finally when it is really healthy, it is not conductive at all. The point is gone, unlike acupuncture points that never disappear.

Auriculotherapy has its practical application in addiction treatment by causing the specific release of neurotransmitters that may be sluggish or in short supply in the addicted brain and spinal cord. The release of these neurotransmitters is stimulated by the application of microcurrent to the nerves in the ear that directly lead into the brain. The electrical current sends a message to increase the activity of the receptor site so that when the neurotransmitter arrives there and places itself in its receptor, the result will be magnified and enhanced. One reason this auriculotherapy is so successful in addiction treatment is that the nerves have direct entry to and from the brain—where the major portion of healing from addiction takes place.

Auriculotherapy is not paint by number. It is always specific to the needs of the individual receiving it. This is made possible because of the precise diagnostic capability of auriculotherapy's microcurrent and specific frequency.

Unlike acupuncture points along meridians, points along the nerves are tangible; you can see them, you can dissect them, and you can measure them. They have a frequency because nerve tissue is tonal. Neurophysiology is very tangible.

The auriculotherapy approach to treatment is clearly defined. It has been found to be safe and effective and the microcurrent instrument has FDA approval. There are hundreds of diseases that auriculotherapy can diagnose and treat, but there are two areas for which it is most successful: pain management and addiction treatment. With pain management it is almost instantaneous; with addiction it is not instantaneous. For addiction recovery there is no quick fix. But this is where auriculotherapy is a plus. It is useful beyond the detoxification stage. Auriculotherapy is usually done initially in recovery after detox in a minimum of ten treatments in a row, five days a week for the first two weeks. We recommend twenty treatments within the first thirty days: five treatments a week.

Auriculotherapy goes beyond the limitations of acu-detox. It can be individualized for each person and for specific drugs and it is a faster procedure. When needles are used, as in acu-detox, they are inserted for forty-five to ninety minutes twice daily. However, needles are inert, do not have frequency or polarity capabilities. Better outcomes can be attained with auriculotherapy in fifteen minutes. With auriculotherapy the skin is not punctured, so treatment is safer.

Dr. Jay Holder and Associates at Exodus Treatment Center in Miami attained a 93 to 96 percent retention rate in residential treatment with the inclusion of auriculartherapy.[5]

Cranial Electrical Stimulation

Since the brain functions by utilizing electrical activity, it follows that mental functions can be influenced by altering the brain's electrical activity. Cranial electrical stimulation (CES) provides a gentle electrical current that stimulates the production of brain chemicals that increase a feeling of wellbeing.[6] CES stimulates the brain by means of two electrodes that are usually placed behind the ear or clipped to the upper portion of the ear lobe. Some clinicians apply the electrodes to the head and the wrist. A pocket-size control unit can be easily carried from place to place.[7]

During CES, an electric current is focused on the hypothalamic region and promotes an increase in endorphins. The current results in an increase of the brain's levels of dopamine, and a decrease in its level of cortisol. When CES is effective, users are in an alert, yet relaxed state, characterized by alpha brain waves.

Electrotherapy has been used for at least 2,000 years, as shown by the clinical literature of the Roman physician Scribonius Largus, who wrote in the *Compositiones Medicae* in 46 AD that his patients should stand on a live black torpedo fish to relieve a variety of medical conditions, including gout and headaches. Modern research into low-intensity electrical stimulation of the brain was begun by Leduc and Rouxeau in France in 1902. In 1949, the Soviet Union expanded CES research to include the treatment of anxiety as well as sleep disorders.

Electrical devices have not caught on until recently. The use of prescription medication to the exclusion of other methods of treating the brain, along with the fear and stigma of using electrical devices on the brain (related to electroconvulsive therapy) has slowed the awareness and acceptance of the effectiveness and safety of electrical stimulation therapy. Public sentiment is beginning to change, however. There is increasing awareness that prescription drugs may not be the safest or most effective way to treat the brain. While CES is still a relatively unknown treatment option, it is gaining recognition for its effectiveness and safety.

Most users of CES report a decrease in anxiety in as little as two days and a noticeable reduction in anxiety within ten treatments. Some (but not all) users report a euphoric feeling. Most report that their thinking is clearer and that they feel more creative.

Studies indicate that low-voltage electrical brain stimulation is therapeutically beneficial in the treatment of conditions such as depression, substance-use disorder, withdrawal symptoms, and insomnia.[8] The FDA has cleared several CES units to be marketed for the treatment of anxiety, depression, and insomnia. There have been no major complications or negative effects associated with CES. A few users feel mild discomfort while using CES but suffer no long-term difficulties.

CES produces an increase in beta-endorphin levels and acetylcholine levels, which blocks anxiety and improves cognitive functioning. It can directly affect the stress levels connected with a reward deficiency in the brain by producing more relaxing, reward-enhancing brain chemistry.

CES has also been shown to significantly improve the P300 brain wave,[9] which has been associated with ADHD as it relates to both drug craving and attention span. Eric Braverman and his associates[10] have shown through brain mapping that many serious brain disorders have electrical rhythm disturbances. CES may normalize a variety of these rhythm disturbances.

Eight

BRAIN-WAVE BIOFEEDBACK (NEUROFEEDBACK)

The nervous system has two major components—voluntary and involuntary. The voluntary component is totally under your control. If you want to move your leg or arm, you simply decide to do it, and your brain does the rest. The brain sends a message, via the nerves, down to the leg, and the leg moves. By contrast, the involuntary nervous system, which controls such body functions as heart rate, blood pressure, and skin temperature, operates out of conscious awareness and without conscious direction from you. However, you can *learn* to control or at least affect many of the involuntary mechanisms, including muscle tension, heart rate, blood supply to the skin, and even emotions.

Biofeedback is a process by which you learn to recognize signals your body provides that tell you how it is functioning. When you weigh yourself or take your heart rate or check your blood pressure, you are receiving feedback from your body about your body.

Body temperature rises as you relax. Do you remember the mood rings that were popular a number of years ago? The ones that changed colors according to your mood? These rings provided a form of biofeedback, changing color as your body temperature changed. The same principle is operating with those stress dots that change color when you put your finger on them. As you relax, the dot or the ring changes color because your body temperature rises.

Mood rings, stress dots, and thermometers are real examples of how we can use biofeedback to have some control over involuntary body functions such as blood pressure, heart rate, and temperature. The more feedback you get, the better able you will be to control involuntary functions on demand and reduce pain, eliminate bad habits, and lower your blood pressure.

Neurofeedback

Neurofeedback (also called brain-wave biofeedback and EEG biofeedback) is a technique by which you train the brain to regulate itself. Neurofeedback allows you to consciously change your mental states by helping you learn to increase or decrease the frequency of your brain waves. It involves displaying a person's brain waves on a computer screen and helping that person learn to control them.

Neurofeedback has a dual role. First, brain waves displayed on a computer monitor can identify when the brain is not functioning well. With the same technology, it is possible to learn to change the brain waves and enable the brain to function better. You can challenge the brain to function better just as you can challenge your muscles to function better with exercise.

Neurofeedback is noninvasive and quite simple. Electrodes are attached to the scalp to monitor brain waves. These electrodes are connected to a computer that supplies feedback as to what is occurring in the brain. Frequency is the rate at which electrical charges move through brain cells. The human brain is measured by four basic frequency ranges.

Delta, the sleep state: very slow brain waves; just 4 cycles (hertz [Hz]) per second.

Theta, a deeply relaxed, daydreaming state, 4 to 8 Hz.

Alpha, a relaxed but alert state, 8 to 13 Hz.

Beta, the most rapid brain waves, reflecting normal waking consciousness in a range from 12 to 35 Hz. (A relaxed but alert state of low beta is 12 to 15 Hz, mid-range beta is 15 to 19 Hz, and an excited, hyper state of high beta can be as high as 35 Hz).

It seems that problems occur when the brain waves are either too slow or too fast. There is speculation that brain-wave frequency may be a major component in a multitude of disorders. The goal of neurofeedback is to stabilize brain-wave frequency. It can be used for closed head injury, post traumatic stress disorder, seizures, sleep disorders, depression, and Tourette's syndrome as well as addiction.. And it can be used by anyone to promote relaxation and a sense of well being and to enhance alertness.

Training Your Brain with Neurofeedback

Two things happen with neurofeedback training. First, you can learn self-regulation, that is, you can learn to alter your own brain waves. You can learn how to speed up the frequency when you need to concentrate and to slow the frequency when you need to relax. Like other types of biofeedback, neurofeedback provides access to our internal processes and allows us to regulate them. The reward of successful self-regulation is the ability to relax if you are highly stressed or the ability to focus if you have trouble concentrating.

Second, with neurofeedback training, actual changes occur in the brain. People who use brain mapping or brain scans report that, as a result of neurofeedback, changes take place in the electrical activity of the brain that persist long term. Deep probes in animal brains have shown that the training has produced actual changes in the brain's neurons.[1] A ten-year study by Joel Lubar of the University of Tennessee at Knoxville and Associates[2] showed that neurofeedback can effectively change what drugs and therapy often can't.

Brain waves are reflective of underlying conditions, an expression of neurotransmitter activity. According to Joel Lubar, neurofeedback increases blood flow into the brain. Blood flow, metabolism, and electrical activity all work together to help the brain reset itself in a normal range. When brain waves are stabilized, symptoms are brought under control. When the problem is slow brain waves, neurofeedback enables the participant to increase beta frequency and be better able to concentrate. When feedback is used to reduce depression, the person can take more responsibility and function better. When the problem is substance use, the desire for the substance diminishes.

Neurofeedback is actually fun and simple for both children and adults. It is like playing a video game. However, instead of controlling the game with your hands you control the activity with your mind. Each time the brain waves find their way into the optimal state set by the practitioner, participants are rewarded with positive feedback. This might be in the form of a Pac Man gobbling up his enemy, a car accelerating, or a pleasant tone or image on the computer monitor. The practitioner sets parameters to be challenging but not too difficult, so that participants can move slowly into their optimal brain states. As they learn to control the signals, they are controlling their own brain-wave patterns. Just like a video game or physical performance, you start at a level that is fairly easy and gradually increase the challenge as your skills increase.

One of the great advantages of neurofeedback over some other neurological interventions is that it can be tailored to each individual. Brain waves can be mapped and analyzed for deviations from the norm. For instance, if there is too much theta—which often occurs in brain trauma, depression, and ADHD—and not enough beta, the practitioner will set parameters to increase beta. After approximately twenty sessions, the brain becomes able to find the optimal state on its own without the help of feedback.

One of the pioneers of neurofeedback was Barry Sterman, professor of neurobiology and biobehavioral psychiatry at the UCLA School of Medicine, who in the '70s used a kind of beta wave called sensory motor rhythm (SMR), in the 12 to 15 Hz range, to treat epilepsy.[3] His original work was on animals. He found that cats and monkeys could be trained to control their brain waves.

After Sterman achieved a 60 percent success rate with humans with even the most severe form of epilepsy, experiments were done at other institutions with even higher success rates.

Beta Training[4]

One of Sterman's researchers, Joel Lubar, noticed that hyperactivity decreased in patients treated for epilepsy; based on this, he created the protocol now used for treatment of ADHD. The protocol is called beta training because ADHD sufferers often show a brain-wave pattern with an excess of theta waves (associated with a day-dreaming state) and a deficit of beta waves (associated with focus and attention). It makes sense, then, that individuals with ADHD are more detached and less focused. With neurofeedback, those with ADHD learn to inhibit their theta waves and enhance their beta waves. It has been regularly demonstrated that with twenty to thirty sessions, people with ADHD can learn to experience greater clarity of thought. Over time these changes have been shown to continue even without further treatments. Joel Lubar claims that more than 90 percent of his patients have benefited.

Merlene Miller, MA and David Miller, PhD

"It Was As If Someone Had Flipped a Switch"

*Beta training was where I started my journey with neurofeedback.
I was curious about the technology. . . . For a half hour or so, I
watched a game: white lines formed in the middle of the highway,
and a beep sounded when I produced the right brain waves. About
an hour after that, it was as if someone had flipped a switch. The
world looked sharp and crystalline, its colors richer. My thinking
was sharper and I had a quiet kind of energy. It lasted a couple of
hours. After five or six sessions, the God-just-painted-the-world effect dissipated, but I noticed other changes. I felt calmer and more
centered. I felt more secure in social situations. Particularly important to me was that my mornings were much more productive. I
always drink coffee and drag my tail until late morning. Lately
I've been getting up, ready to go. By the fifteenth session, the change
was unmistakable. As of th is writing, it has lasted about a month.*

Jim Robbins

ALPHA-THETA PROTOCOL[6]

The alpha-theta protocol is very different from beta training. It takes
place in the lower registers of the brain's frequencies. The first study of
the effectiveness of the alpha-theta protocol on substance abusers was
begun in 1982 by Eugene Peniston, a researcher at the Sam Rayburn
Memorial Veterans' Center in Bonham, Texas. Peniston hypothesized
that alcoholics drink because they cannot get into alpha states naturally, and therefore, cannot produce soothing neurotransmitters on their
own. He compared ten alcoholics treated with traditional counseling
with ten others who had the same counseling plus the alpha-theta
training. Peniston claims an 80 percent success rate with those who
used the neurofeedback—compared to 20 percent for those receiving
traditional treatment.

Memory Training

Scientists from Imperial College, London, and Charing Cross Hospital have announced[7] that they have been able to improve working memory by 10 percent with neurofeedback training. Working memory is a type of memory used to hold and then apply information to perform a task, such as holding a phone number in your mind to recall and use later. The ability to improve working memory is good news for recovering addicts with memory problems.

We should note here that neurofeedback is not a method for detoxification. You should be through withdrawal before using it. We would also caution you to work with a practitioner who identifies your specific brain-wave patterns to determine the type of protocol most appropriate for you.

There are critics of neurofeedback who say that any benefits are due to a placebo effect, but animal studies show that placebo cannot be the primary reason that brain-wave biofeedback is effective. Why not? Because placebos do not work on animals. Of course, there is always the possibility of placebo effects in human studies. Expectancy does produce a reaction. But the practitioner can switch around protocols and get different results. (False feedback does not produce the same effect as accurate feedback.) This would not be the case with a placebo effect. Because the participant is not able to tell when the practitioner switches protocols and would not respond because of expectation.

Whether you have a specific disorder such as ADHD or just want to improve the functioning of your brain, neurofeedback can be beneficial. When your brain functions better, you will sleep better, you will feel more serene, you will be able to manage your focus and attention, and you will feel more emotionally stable.

Nine

BODY WORK

There are a variety of body therapies that you might find beneficial in recovery for natural pain relief, relieving stress, increasing energy, and lifting your mood. Many touch therapies are becoming more and more popular as the benefits become better known. Any of the following methods of balancing or relaxing body tissue can enhance comfort in sobriety.

Therapeutic Massage

Therapeutic massage is used for both relieving pain and reducing stress. In fact, it is based on the idea that there is a relationship between muscle pain and stress; that is, relaxing muscles reduces stress, and reducing stress relaxes muscles. The added benefit is that, when stress responses are lowered, physical disorders, such as high blood pressure and diabetes, improve. Therapeutic massage—sometimes referred to as Swedish massage—originated about 5,000 years ago in

Sweden, thus it's passed the test of time as a way to improve health and wellbeing.

Reiki and Therapeutic Touch

Reiki and Therapeutic Touch are techniques concerned with moving energy through the body to restore balance. They are based on the idea that there are energy fields within and around the body. These techniques are intended to balance and restore harmony throughout the energy system of the body.

Reiki originated in Japan as a way to bring the mind, body, and spirit into balance. It came from a technique described in Tibetan scriptures almost 3,000 years ago. Therapeutic Touch is the work of Dora Kuntz and Delores Krieger and is influenced by yoga and the Ayurvedic, Tibetan, and Chinese health systems.

With both techniques, there may or may not be physical contact between the therapist and the client; however, Reiki is usually a hands-on procedure and Therapeutic Touch is usually hands off. Therapeutic Touch is usually done with the hand about four inches above the body. It is sometimes said that Reiki allows the energy flow and Therapeutic Touch directs the energy flow.

Therapeutic Touch includes an assessment during which the therapist identifies blockages in energy flow by a feeling of coldness; infection or excess energy by a feeling of warmth; and congestion by variations in sensations experienced. The practitioner works with the client until these areas all feel similar—no area is hotter, colder, or more congested than another. The average treatment lasts about twenty minutes .

Research has discovered that Reiki and Therapeutic Touch offer similar benefits: relaxation, decreased anxiety, increased sense of well-being, and healing. Both have been found to have a calming effect and to decrease anxiety. When nurses use therapeutic touch, patients have been found to need less pain medication.

Reflexology

Reflexology is a micro-system therapy; that is, various points on the feet are thought to represent various organs and parts of the body. Reflexologists claim that work on these points improves blood flow and energy, thus improving functioning in the corresponding part of the body. Tenderness at a specific site on the foot indicates a potential problem in the associated part of the body. Pressure on that spot leads to unblocked energy.

During a reflexology session, the therapist applies gentle but firm pressure or massage to your feet. Like a good massage, reflexology is very relaxing and is said to lessen anxiety. It is generally safe, but you should still take some precautions. For example, if your feet have been injured in any way, postpone treatment until they've healed. Most reflexologists will not treat you if you have a fever; if you've recently had surgery; if you have any vascular problem in your lower legs; or if you have a pacemaker. So long as you follow these precautions and do not rely on reflexology for any diagnostic purposes, it appears to be a safe way to decrease tension and relieve pain.

Rolfing

Rolfing, developed by biophysicist Ida Rolf, focuses on the fascia, or connective tissue that binds and connects the body's bones and muscles. Normal fascia is loose, moist, and mobile, allowing muscles and joints to move easily and remain flexible. Chronic stress, injury, and inactivity cause the fascia to thicken and its layers to fuse together.

The purpose of Rolfing is to stretch and unwind the thickened fascia, reestablish proper alignment, restoring the normal relationship between bones and muscles, and improve their function. Rolfers claim to be able to reduce pain and spasms, raise your energy levels, improve mood, and make the body more limber, and increase range of motion in the joints.

Myofascial Release

As the name implies, myofascial release also focuses on connective tissue. It is based on the idea that when the myofascia is damaged the constrictions and restrictions interfere with proper functioning throughout the body. When these constrictions are released, there is not only physical relief but also emotional and mental release. Although there are few studies to support myofascial release, it is rapidly becoming more popular, and many who experience it report dramatic outcomes.

Merlene: *Because I had a daughter-in-law who was a massage therapist that practiced myofascial release, I had heard quite a bit about the therapy's benefits and many stories of astounding outcomes. I had a couple of treatments and then decided to get what is called an intensive—about 100 hours in three weeks from a therapist in my area. It was an amazing experience. Something happens with myofascial release that I have not heard about with other forms of massage—involuntary movement. The therapist massages one part of the body, and another part moves. I don't mean this is involuntary movement in the sense that I couldn't stop it but in the sense that I didn't consciously initiate it. And I* *usually did not attempt to stop it because I did not feel at risk in any way. If I did, I could have stopped it. Sometimes it felt as if I had large strands of taffy inside and someone was pulling the taffy on one end causing a response at the point where it was connected at the other end. After I was comfortable with what was happening to me I was able to relax and just let it happen, often entering a very relaxed state in which I had a sense of enlightenment and awareness. At the end of my intensive, I felt better physically, mentally, and spiritually than I can remember feeling since I was a child. I had much more freedom of movement; I felt clean mentally and emotionally; and my energy level was increased.*

The Rosen Method

The Rosen Method is a therapy developed by Martha Rosen that combines massage with a form of nondirective counseling. It is based on the idea that traumas and memories are stored in the body as muscular tension. Agitated emotions often result in tense muscles and those emotions can be released through massage. As the massage moves to various areas of the body, the therapist—while monitoring breathing and asking questions—gets the client to talk about potential emotional blocks. The combination of massage and discussion can bring memories and emotions to the surface. Often awareness of the emotion is therapeutic; in other instances, talking about the emotions is helpful.

Shiatsu

Shiatsu originated in Japan about seventy years ago and is based on Chinese medicine practice. It is considered massage but it is really more a form of acupressure. Like acupuncture, it targets the points where energy flows along meridians throughout the body. It is credited with bringing about the same types of results as acupuncture: primarily pain relief and relaxation.

Craniosacral Therapy

Cerebrospinal fluid bathes the brain and the tissues of the spinal cord. It is prevented from leaking out into the rest of the body by a membrane that encloses the entire nervous system. Cerebrospinal fluid normally flows freely from the head (cranium) to the base of the spine (sacrum). According to craniosacral therapists, this nervous system circulation has a rhythm of its own. They theorize that anything that interrupts the normal flow of cerebrospinal fluid or alters its rhythm and pressure can cause physical and mental problems.

William Sutherland, an osteopath, formulated the theory of craniosacral therapy in the early 1900s. During the last twenty years, his work has been continued and popularized by another osteopathic physician, John Upledger. In the late 1970s, Upledger headed a team of scientists at Michigan State University that produced a model demonstrating the movement of fluid in the nervous system from the head to the tailbone. The researchers concluded that the craniosacral system acts like a semi-closed hydraulic system. Anything that interferes with the flow of spinal fluid flow prevents this movement and raises the pressure on the membranes as well as the tissues of the brain or the spinal cord. This can result in pain from your head to your tail, as well as emotional and behavioral problems. Craniosacral therapy is intended to relieve the pressure that interferes with the flow of spinal fluid with gentle pressure to the bones of the skull.

Ten

Essential Oil Therapy

For thousands of years, humankind has benefited from the healing properties of plant oils. Incense and aromatic oils have been used for millennia to enhance religious rituals, to embalm bodies, and to mask unpleasant odors. It wasn't until the 1920s, though, that essential oil therapy became a formal discipline within health care.

Essential oils are aromatic substances extracted from various plant parts including flowers, roots, bark, leaves, wood resins, and citrus rinds. Essential oils can be sprayed into the air and inhaled or absorbed through the skin via massage, hot baths, or hot or cold compresses. Some essential oils can be taken internally, but we do not recommend this because a few are toxic when ingested. Essential oils are extracted in concentrated form, but by the time you buy them they have been combined with other carrier oils in order to be used safely.

Essential oils improve your mood and promote good health. Some soothe, some relax, some stimulate and invigorate. They work by reacting with hormones and enzymes after they enter the bloodstream. Essential oils may affect your pulse, blood pressure,

Merlene Miller, MA and David Miller, PhD

or evoke specific memories. For example, clove, rosemary, lavender, and mint stimulate the salivary glands; camphor, calamus, and hyssop are good for the heart and circulation; other aromatics act on the lymphatic, endocrine, nervous, and urinary systems; and bergamot, lavender, and juniper have antiseptic properties, and are said to help a variety of dermatologic disorders when applied to the skin.

> ## "To His Surprise, the Pain and Redness Subsided Very Quickly"
>
> It happened serendipitously when René-Maurice Gattefossé, a French chemist working in the perfume industry, burned his hand very badly. The only "therapy" immediately available to him was a container of pure lavender oil into which he plunged his scorched hand. To his surprise, the pain and redness subsided very quickly, and Gattefossé claimed that the burn healed within hours without leaving a scar. The chemist attributed this salutary effect to the healing and antiseptic properties of the lavender oil. He experimented with several other oils and decided that they, too, had potential for healing a variety of skin disorders. Other French physicians, notably Dr. Jean Valnet, began to use aromatic oils not only for skin problems but for other medical disorders as well, such as anxiety and insomnia. Valnet, who served as an army surgeon during World War II, treated burns and other wounds with essential oils such as clove, thyme, and chamomile. He also found that certain fragrances alleviated some psychiatric problems.
>
> From *Dr. Rosenfeld's Guide to Alternative Medicine*[1]

Calming and comforting oils include sage, sandalwood, patchouli, thyme, jasmine, chamomile, oregano, marjoram, and lavender. Sesquiterpenes, found in the oils of frankincense and sandalwood, help increase the amount of oxygen in the limbic system of the brain, leading to an increase in opioids. Lavender is one of the most popular plants in essential oil therapy. It is known for its relaxing and calming effects, and it is also an excellent remedy for headaches and insomnia. For gentle relaxation, try soaking a towel in warm water infused with lavender. You can re-warm the towel in a microwave and bring the lavender scent to your face and hands to experience this aromatic relaxation.

Invigorating herbal oils include mountain savory, peppermint, spearmint, ginger, citrus, mint, and cardamom. Oils that promote clarity of thought are petitgrain, rosemary, cedarwood, basil, spruce, ginger, fir, bergamot, and clove. Oils that are emotionally healing include cypress, eucalyptus, and wild tansy. Oils that increase spiritual awareness and promote emotional harmony and balance are frankincense, galbanum, grapefruit, melissa, myrrh, yarrow, and juniper. To improve sleep, try chamomile, lavender, or marjoram.

Inhalation

Pleasant aromas can lift your mood, help you sleep, and aid in relaxation. When we inhale a particular scent, it is picked up by two small patches of tissue in the nasal cavity that contain more than 20 million nerve endings that are stimulated by aromas. The scent is converted into a nerve message that is immediately transmitted to the limbic system of the brain, which then relays the aroma to the hypothalamus, triggering both emotional and physiological responses.

A good way to get the most benefit from herbs and flowers is by extracting the essence of the plant by steeping it in water or oil. You can do this yourself using small jars with tight-fitting lids. (Do not use plastic containers). Place two large handfuls of herbs or flowers in a saucepan. Use a neutrally flavored vegetable oil to cover the herbs or flowers. Heat at a low temperature for twenty to thirty minutes, let the oil cool, strain it into a jar, close tightly, and store in a cool, dark place for up to three weeks. To fill a room with the aroma, place the opened jar on a table. (You can also pour some oil in your bath water or rub it on your body after a bath or shower)[2]

To prevent inhaling the oil, take care when using a diffuser with essential oil. Certain oils must be used with caution as they are known allergens. Too much of any type of oil might result in an abnormal response. Rosemary appears to have a blood sugar–raising effect. Eucalyptus citriodora has been found to have a blood sugar–lowering effect.

Topical Application

Oils can be applied directly to the skin, typically using one to six drops of oil. One to three drops are usually adequate. Oil placed on the feet is rapidly absorbed because of large pores. The ears and the wrists will also rapidly absorb oils. If you are massaging oil onto a large area of the body, dilute the oil by about 30 percent with a neutral-smelling vegetable oil. Don't try to create your own blends of essential oils. Commercial blends are available that have been formulated by people who understand the chemical nature of each oil and how they blend. If mixed improperly, their chemical properties can be altered and you can get an undesirable reaction. It is better to layer individual oils: apply one oil at a time, rub it in, and then apply another oil.

What Science Says About Essential Oils

Here is what some scientifically valid studies report on the benefits of aromas:

Sleep: In a 1995 report in *The Lancet,* elderly patients who required substantial doses of sleeping pills slept like babies when a lavender aroma was wafted into their bedrooms at night.

Behavior: Mice made hyper-excitable by large amounts of caffeine were calmed by fragrances of lavender, sandalwood, and other oils sprayed into their cages. On the other hand, they became more irritable when exposed to the aroma of orange terpenes, thymol, and certain other substances.

Stress: At Memorial Sloan-Kettering Hospital in New York, after exposure to the aroma of vanilla, patients reported that they were 63 percent less claustrophobic. The patients' anxiety may have been lessened by the intensity of the pleasant memories evoked by the vanilla aroma. In another study of 122 patients under obvious stress in an intensive care unit, patients felt much better when they were given aromatherapy with oil of lavender than when they simply rested or had a massage.

Isadore Rosenfeld, MD[3]

Oils and Water

Essential oils mixed with water can be very pleasing and relaxing. You can fill a water basin with hot water, stir in essential oils, and lay a towel on top of the water to make a compress. The oils will float to the top, so the towel will absorb the oils in the water. After the towel is completely saturated, wring it out and place it over the area of your body needing the compress. Or you can add three to six drops of oil to your bath water while the tub is filling. Your skin will quickly draw the oil from the top of the water as you soak for about fifteen minutes. Or you can add three to six drops of oil to a half-ounce of bath or shower gel base and add it to your bath water. When showering, you can add three to six drops of oil to a bath or shower gel and apply it to a washcloth.

Raindrop Therapy

Gary Young, of Young Essential Oils, an aromatologist and expert on the art and science of aromatherapy, has developed an application technique called raindrop therapy. This involves dropping oils directly onto the spine from about six inches above the body. The oils are worked into the spine with light strokes that stimulate energy impulses and disperse the oil along the nervous system. This is believed to bring the body into balance. A raindrop massage lasts about forty-five minutes, but the oils continue to work in the body for a week or more following the therapy. Oils used in raindrop therapy are Valor (a blend of rosewood, blue tansy, frankincense, and spruce), thyme, oregano, cypress, birch, basil, peppermint, marjoram, and Aroma Siez (a blend of basil, lavender, cypress, and marjoram).

Vita Flex Therapy

Vita Flex Therapy, part of a system developed by Stanley Burroughs, uses the reflex system of the body to release tension. It combines using essential oils with a form of massage similar to reflexology for the whole body. Applied with rotation hand movements, the massage releases healing energy along the neuro-electrical pathways. Healing energy is created by the contact between the fingertips and contact points. The resulting energy follows the neuro-pathways of the nervous system to points where there is a break in the electrical circuit. This technique is believed to have originated in Tibet, many thousands of years ago, before acupuncture was discovered. Vita Flex therapists say this is a superior form of reflexology.

Although it utilizes the same principles, Vita Flex produces less discomfort than traditional reflexology. In addition, there are 5,000 identified Vita Flex points in the body, compared to 365 acupuncture points used in reflexology. Combining the electrical energy with the healing properties of essential oils releases healing power, relieving tension, drowsiness, weariness, and discomfort. Oils used in Vita Flex Therapy are Valor and White Angelica (a blend of ylang ylang, rose, angelica, melissa, sandalwood, geranium, spruce, myrrh, hyssop, bergamot, and rosewood).

If you are considering essential oil therapy, or are already using it, there are certain cautions you should take. According to Isadore Rosenfeld, MD:

- Aromatic oils vary in quality, and their production is not regulated, so make sure your source is reliable. Always ask for the purest available brand.
- Do not consume aromatic oils. Some can be toxic.
- Store aromatic oils in a cool place. Some, such as jasmine and neroli, should be refrigerated. Most oils retain their potency for two to three years, but citrus oils lose their potency within a year.
- With the exception of topical lavender oil for burns or insect bites, never use concentrated, undiluted oil. Refer to a good book on aromatherapy for instructions on diluting oil.

- If your skin is sensitive, always apply a very small amount of the diluted oil before you try the whole treatment, to make sure you're not allergic to it. Five percent of the population reacts adversely to aromatic oils.
- Keep all aromatic oils away from children.
- Always close your eyes when inhaling aromatic oil. The vapors can be irritating at close range. Don't apply any oils close to your eyes.
- Do not use mint oils at night—they can cause insomnia.
- Avoid oils of sweet fennel and rosemary if you have epilepsy. These substances may increase the excitability of the brain and induce seizures.
- If you're pregnant, avoid oils of arnica, basil, clary sage, cypress, juniper, myrrh, sage, and thyme. Some obstetricians believe that these oils can cause the uterus to contract. A woman who is at risk of a miscarriage, or who has abnormal bleeding, should keep away from chamomile and lavender. If the doctor approves, a pregnant woman may use diluted oils of peppermint, rose, and rosemary after the fourth month.
- People with high blood pressure should avoid oils of rosemary, sage, and thyme.

Eleven

SUPPORT PEOPLE

A successful recovery involves developing new and more meaningful social networks. That means finding resources and making contacts that will enable you to meet new people who can offer more than just drinking company. As you replace drug use with meaningful, enduring values and activities, you will want to associate with people who share those values.

They say in AA that to find sobriety you must change playgrounds and playmates. The people you associated with while using are tied to your addiction-based lifestyle. It is not that they are bad; you just have one central thing in common with them—your use of mood-altering substances. If you choose to spend most of your time around old using buddies, ignoring their expectations for you to use chemicals can become stressful or even impossible.

As for the playgrounds, it has been said that no one frequents a house of ill repute to listen to the piano player. By the same token, you do not go to a bar to have orange juice. It is not just a question of not associating with your old friends or not frequenting your old hangouts. It is more a question of what new places you are going to and what new friends you are meeting. Your playgrounds will change automatically as you meet new sober people.

Being a social animal is different from being a party animal. Becoming social is an art; being a party animal is nothing more than getting high or drunk, laughing a lot, acting crazy, and not remembering what you did or said. Reorienting your lifestyle around new values is an essential part of recovery. The values that allowed you to keep using will not allow you to stay sober. A lifestyle conducive to using is not conducive to sobriety. Friends who encourage drinking or using do not usually encourage abstinence. Places where it was easy to drink or use are not usually places where it is easy not to. New friends, new activities, and new social contacts are part of recovery.

Mutual-Help Groups

A mutual-help group is a valuable source for establishing or reestablishing a meaningful social network. You will find people that understand not only your struggles but your need for deeper and more meaningful relationships. They will offer you friendship, support, acceptance, and encouragement. They provide fun activities without alcohol or other drugs. Don't forget how important it is to learn to have fun—with people who do not center their good times around mood-altering chemicals.

In recovery, you need the support of others, especially the support of people with the same condition. For those who have problems relating to the principles or practices of twelve step groups there are other support groups available. Most groups—whether twelve step or another group—encourage a new way of life based on honesty and reaching out to others. They offer a means for making the right changes at the right time. They are based on members sharing their experiences and what has worked for them. These groups are places where you can meet people with whom you can feel safe and comfortable in new and healthy ways as you attempt to understand the disorder you have and share with those in the same boat.

ALCOHOLICS ANONYMOUS

The most well-known support group is Alcoholics Anonymous (AA), founded in the 1930s by people who had tried many other methods of abstaining from alcohol and had failed. They found that mutual support enabled them to do what had previously been unattainable. AA has endured over the years, and its principles apply to other twelve-step programs such as Narcotics Anonymous, Overeaters Anonymous, Cocaine Anonymous, and Gamblers Anonymous.

AA is especially helpful for individuals who prefer a spiritually-based group. The steps of AA are spiritual principles. AA encourages you to accept the help of a higher power, though that power can be defined as you choose. It can even be the power of the group itself.

AA offers the recovering person much that professional treatment cannot offer. It offers a readily available environment that is conducive to ongoing recovery and sobriety. AA is available twenty-four hours a day in every major city around the world. You are never farther away from a meeting than the telephone. In large metropolitan areas, meetings are held at all times of the day and night. You can always have the phone number of someone who will help you avoid that one drinking or drug episode.

AA doesn't cost anything except time, energy, and a motivation to stop drinking or using. You need a place to go to meet other people who want to have fun and socialize without drugs or alcohol. Many recovering people begin rebuilding their social life with friends and acquaintances they find at meetings.

RATIONAL RECOVERY

Rational recovery (RR) is an alternative support program utilized primarily by people who are uncomfortable with the spiritual nature of Alcoholics Anonymous. As the name implies, RR is based on the concepts of rational thinking. It was started by Jack Trimpey using the principles of rational-emotive therapy developed by Albert Ellis. In rational recovery, you learn to be aware of your emotions and where they come from. You learn to recognize that emotions are not forced upon you by others or by outside situations. They are your own response to situations, and you can learn to control your response. Rational recovery suggests the five-point criteria developed by Maxie Maultsby to evaluate a thought to determine whether it is logical.

1. If I believe this thought to be true, will it help me remain sober, safe, and alive?
2. Is this thought objectively true, and upon what evidence am I forming this opinion?
3. Is this thought producing feelings I want to have?
4. Is this thought helping me reach a chosen goal?
5. Is this thought likely to minimize conflict with others?

Rational recovery helps you identify irrational ideas and beliefs that perpetuate addictive behavior and then provides the means to change your emotions and behavior.[1]

An AA Sponsor

The principles of AA are simple, but at first they can be misunderstood. Therefore, a practice has developed whereby experienced members make themselves available to newer members as a sponsor. A sponsor's responsibility is to provide support during recovery, answer questions, discuss the various aspects of the program, assist the new members in identifying meetings that meet their needs, and direct them to appropriate literature and resources that they may need to fully understand the program.

AA sponsors are not therapists or counselors, nor are they responsible for telling other members how to work their programs. All members are responsible for interpreting the principles for themselves and developing their own programs based on those principles. The sponsor is merely a sounding board, a supportive friend, and a knowledgeable resource.

Counseling

If you started drinking or using drugs early in life, you may have skipped some developmental stages of growth. The teens and early twenties are years when emotional and social maturation take place. If drinking and drug use occur during that time, that developmental process may not occur or it may be retarded.

At whatever point you are ready to give up drug or alcohol use as a way of coping with life, counseling can aid you in the process of learning to manage your emotions and developing the insights and self-awareness that you may have missed by addictive living.

A counselor can help you resolve the pervasive shame that may affect your recovery. Addiction is often accompanied by shame for a number of reasons. First you may feel shame because of a condition that existed before your addiction (such as ADHD) and which increased your vulnerability for using mood-altering substances. Second, you may have done things while drinking or using drugs that you would not do sober and which are very shameful to you now. Third, you may have a history of repeated relapse that you and other people interpret as being weak willed or lacking strength of character. (Actually, the fact that you have kept trying despite what has been perceived as failure shows strong will and strength of character.) And fourth, there is the stigma that accompanies addiction. Our society views addiction as a shameful condition. Even though we live in a culture that encourages drinking, overeating, pill popping, and other excesses, when a person becomes addicted to alcohol, pills, food, or gambling, they are looked upon as morally lacking, self-centered, pleasure-obsessed individuals. Learning to accept yourself as a person of worth despite the burden of shame that you or society has placed upon you can be a positive outcome of counseling. A counselor can help you replace misperceptions you may have about yourself, the world, or your addiction with accurate perceptions that facilitate behavior change.

In recovery you may need to learn or relearn certain life skills. If you want to change your behavior, a counselor can help. You have developed many skills that have helped you survive addiction. These same skills can be modified to help you live sober.

David: *I am a reality therapist. I like reality therapy (RT) because it is a very simple approach to helping you change your behavior. It asks you some direct questions to help you evaluate what you are doing and help you make plans to change what you are doing if you really want to change. The questions are: What are you doing now? Is that working for you? If not, what are you going to do instead? The idea is to figure out what is not working in your life and not just eliminate it but replace it with a better chosen behavior. With RT you take small, manageable steps that lead you where you want to go.*

Coaching

Coaching is not counseling. Coaching is a term taken from sports that refers to an alliance that empowers success. Coaching is now being used to empower professional success, educational success, and personal success. ADHD coaching is being used extensively by people with attention deficit hyperactivity disorder. We recommend ADHD-type coaching for people recovering from addiction. In the first place, many of you who have had problems with addiction also have attention deficit disorder, treated or untreated. Second, people in sobriety experience many of the symptoms of ADHD. Third, and most important, many of the skills that people with ADHD need to develop are lacking in those with addictions.

The purpose of any coaching is to enhance performance. The purpose of ADHD coaching is to enable you to enhance performance by helping you (1) set goals, (2) devise a plan for reaching your goals, (3) set priorities, (4) make decisions, and (5) keep on track. A coach offers guidance and support while giving responsibility to you

The first phase in the coaching process is setting the agenda—identifying your long-term goals. And remember, this is your agenda, not the coach's agenda. The second phase is making short-term goals that will meet day-to-day needs and help you achieve your long-term goals. During the second phase, it is important to review your progress to determine if the long-term goals are still applicable.

The value of coaching is having someone available to guide you when you find it difficult to sort things out and prioritize tasks. Someone trained to do so can help you keep on track by continually holding up your goals and identifying whether your actions will achieve your goals. The coach can help you keep moving when you feel paralyzed by the obstacles you encounter as you face the problems created by your addiction.

The coach can also help you: identify what supports need to be put in place to increase your chances for success, determine what you want or need to accomplish between coaching sessions, and decide what tasks will help you accomplish those things. When you and the coach determine what skills are lacking that prevent you from achieving your goals, you will make plans for developing those skills or change your goals according to the skills you already have. The greatest value of having a coach is having someone to provide regular reminders of where you want to go and what you need to do to get there.

Coaching differs from counseling in that the power lies not in the coach or the client but in the coaching alliance. The client is a full partner in the alliance. The coach's goal is always to facilitate the client's agenda. By asking powerful and direct questions, reminding you of your agenda, and keeping you focused, the coach allows you to plan your own course and take the steps to keep you on it.

The alliance provides a safe environment for you to practice developing life skills, continually holding up your goals and identifying whether your actions will achieve your goals. The coach can help you keep moving when you feel paralyzed by the obstacles you encounter as you face the problems created by your addiction. The coach can also help you: identify what supports need to be put in place to increase your chances for success, determine what you want or need to accomplish between coaching sessions, and decide what tasks will help you accomplish those things. When you and the coach determine what skills are lacking that prevent you from achieving your goals, you will make plans for developing those skills or change your goals according to the skills you already have. The greatest value of having a coach is having someone to provide regular reminders of where you want to go and what you need to do to get there.

Twelve

STRESS-REDUCING ACTIVITIES

Stress affects your body and your mind. It affects your thinking, feelings, memory, sleep patterns, daily functioning, and physical and mental health. When a sudden alert is sounded in the body, the center part of the brain, or the hypothalamus, sends a message to the adrenal gland to release cortisol. Cortisol increases the heart rate, increases the blood pressure, and releases stored glucose from the liver and muscle cells into the bloodstream for quick energy.

Some stress in life is necessary. It keeps you functioning. Without some stress you would not take care of yourself, go to work, or do anything for your family. But too much stress is harmful. Each of us has a level of stress at which we function most effectively. Your best stress level is high enough to keep you productive, yet low enough not to hurt you or the people around you. Finding the level of stress that is useful without being destructive is important for your recovery from addiction. You can relapse because of too little stress (no constructive concern about your addiction) or because of too much stress (which produces excessive worry and anxiety).

One of the most agonizing chronic abstinence symptoms is stress sensitivity. Most recovering people have a low stress tolerance and overreact to stress. As we have discussed before, this can sabotage even the best efforts at sobriety. We have talked about foods and supplements and environmental changes to reduce stress levels. There are also actions you can take to reduce stress and increase serenity and peace of mind. The relaxation response (the decrease of blood pressure and pulse rate and the improved utilization of oxygen) occurs because of what you do and think. You can learn to relax.

Deep Relaxation

You are probably aware that your muscles cannot relax and tense at the same time. You can learn to relax your muscles when you choose, thereby reducing tension. You can also learn to form pictures in your mind that help you relax. And you can learn to talk to yourself in a way that reduces tension and increases your feelings of comfort and well-being.

Deep relaxation allows the body and mind to reduce stress and produce a sense of well-being. What occurs when you relax is the opposite of what is called the fight or flight response. When you relax, your muscles become heavy, your body temperature rises, and your breathing and heart rate slow down.

To experience deep relaxation, create a quiet place for yourself. Separate yourself from the world in your quiet place. Lie on your back or sit in a comfortable chair with your feet on the floor. Close your eyes, release distracting thoughts, try to put background noises and sounds out of your thoughts. Breathe deeply and relax your body. You do not make your body relax—you allow it to relax. You focus your concentration on one thing and allow distractions to drift from your awareness.

With some relaxation methods, the focus is on the physical states you are trying to change (your muscles, body temperature, breathing, or heartbeat). With other methods, you do not concentrate on your physical state, but on a color, a sound, a word or mantra, or a mental image.

If you choose to focus on physical states, begin with your muscles. Allow them to become heavy. Then concentrate on raising your temperature. You can do this by sensing a spot of heat in your forehead or chest and allowing it to flow throughout your body. Then think about your breathing. Let it become slower and slower. Breathe from your abdomen, rather than your chest. Then feel your heartbeat and concentrate on slowing it down.

If you choose to relax by concentrating on something other than your physical state, you can think of a color. Concentrate on that color, fill your mind with that color, become a part of that color. Or feel yourself in motion, floating, tumbling, and rolling. Or repeat a pleasant word over and over to yourself. Or imagine yourself in a soothing place, such as by a quiet lake, in a green meadow, or in a beautiful garden. These are relaxation exercises you can do by yourself without the aid of a book or a tape.

Numerous books and tapes are available to guide you through the relaxation process. Or you can record a tape yourself and play it when you want to relax. Deep relaxation reduces your stress and helps you feel better. Relaxation exercises can help you manage chronic abstinence symptoms and heal your addicted brain.

Breathing

Deep breathing aids in relaxation. In his newsletter, "Self- Healing, "Dr. Andrew Weil has noted that deep breathing has been shown to lower blood pressure, decrease or stop heart arrhythmias, improve digestion, increase blood circulation, decrease anxiety, and improve the quality of sleep. To distinguish deep breathing from shallow breathing, pay attention to your chest and your abdomen. Chest breathing is usually shallow breathing; abdominal breathing is usually deep breathing. Dr. Weil describes a yoga-style method of breathing like this:

Start by sitting with your back straight or lying in a comfortable position. Place the tip of your tongue to the ridge in back of your upper front teeth and keep it there during the entire exercise. Exhale through the mouth with a whoosh sound. Close your mouth and inhale through your nose to the count of four. Hold your breath for seven counts and then exhale, with the whoosh sound, to the count of eight. Do this for four cycles.

There is a connection between your breathing and your emotional state. Fear, anger, and frustration restrict breathing. Restricted breathing increases negative emotional states. Your sense of well-being can be enhanced by your breathing. When you calm your breath you calm your mind. Calming your breathing throughout the day brings a sense of peacefulness. The constitution of the blood is altered through oxygen exchange which, in turn, leads to more relaxed breathing. Here is another deep breathing exercise you can try:

While sitting or lying down, place your hands on your stomach or chest.

Sigh (audibly) several times.

Slowly and fully inhale through the mouth, filling your lungs comfortably from the bottom to the top. Imagine you are bringing energy into your body.

Without hesitation, exhale through your nose, emptying your lungs from the top to the bottom comfortably. Visualize yourself releasing your tensions as you breathe out.

Repeat this procedure for ten to fifteen minutes, until you are totally and pleasantly absorbed with the breathing process and alert but not focusing on any other thoughts or activities. There will be a feeling of peace and serenity just in controlling your breathing process.

Yoga

Developed over centuries, yoga is used to reduce stress, improve flexibility, and provide mental clarity. Yoga is a technique with three major components: posture, breathing, and meditation. The first objective of yoga is to maintain one of a variety of yoga poses for a specified period of time. The ultimate goal is to gain the self control needed for proper breathing and for effective meditation. The breathing exercises consist of a routine in which the lungs are filled with air that is held and then released.

The goal of the meditation component is to detach from your environment and to experience peace, enlightenment, and tranquility. Here is a scaled-down version of yoga that you can follow easily and effectively, as described in the "Lifetime Health Letter"[1] from the University of Texas-Houston.

For exercise: Sit forward in a chair, your feet flat on the floor. Put your right hand on your left knee. With your left hand, hold the back of the chair. Look straight ahead, inhale, and then as you slowly exhale, turn to your left. Pull with both hands to rotate your spine as much as possible without strain. Hold the rotated position for a few seconds, continuing to breathe easily. Return to the forward position. Then, put your left hand on your right knee, and repeat the steps, twisting to the right.

For breathing: Sit straight with both hands flat against your stomach, just below the navel. Relax your stomach and allow it to push out as you inhale. Then, as you exhale, tighten your stomach and flatten your back. Concentrate on the sound your breath makes in the back of your throat. Breathe smoothly and steadily through your nose; don't hold your breath at any time. Repeat this procedure several times.

For meditation: Sit quietly and comfortably in a chair or on the floor. Close your eyes and take a few full, deep breaths. Concentrate on the sound you make when you breathe in and out. Relax your breath and, at the same time, consciously relax your facial muscles. Progressively relax the rest of your body, beginning with the shoulders and arms, working your way down to your feet. Become limp without slouching. Try to be completely silent, inside and out. Imagine a pleasant scene to help yourself achieve total relaxation. After a few minutes, begin to breathe more deeply; then stretch your arms and imagine your energy being totally renewed.

Several scientific reports suggest that yoga can reduce blood pressure and heart rate and improve circulation, as well as help you relax, ease chronic pain, and improve your memory and concentration. Some of these benefits may be due to a release of opioids.

Sleep

Sleep is an important ingredient of good health. Because of your addictive lifestyle, you may have developed poor sleep habits. In addition, you may experience abstinence-related sleep problems. This may be especially true if you have used alcohol excessively in the past. Although alcohol is sedating, it disrupts normal sleep patterns and deprives you of REM sleep (dream sleep). When you are no longer drinking, there is a rebound effect in which your body tries to catch up on lost REM sleep and, for a period of time, you may experience an excessive amount of disturbing dreams.

To enhance the quality of recovery, you may need to enhance the quality and quantity of sleep. The following are some general considerations:

- Be sure the temperature of the room is comfortable for you. Wear socks to bed if you have cold feet.
- Maintain regular sleeping times by going to sleep and awakening at the same time each day.
- Avoid exercising close to bedtime. Exercise is a stimulant and can disturb your sleep.
- Avoid stimulants such as caffeine (or tyrosine) near bedtime.
- Take a warm bath or shower close to bedtime.
- Begin to relax and wind down beginning two hours before bedtime: Listen to music. Do relaxation exercises. Read.
- Eat a high complex carbohydrate dinner with little or no protein.
- Eat a high-tryptophan bedtime snack.
- Choose your mattress and pillows carefully. Make sure your weight is evenly distributed. Make sure your pillow provides enough support for your neck.
- Maintain a quiet bedroom without bright lights.

Physical Exercise

We have a friend who used to say, "I have a theory that exercise causes cancer. The only thing I exercise is caution. I only enjoy long walks when they are taken by people who nag me to exercise." She was kidding, of course, but behind the humor she was saying something many people would like to say, "We would like a good excuse not to exercise and any good theory will do." The interesting thing we want you to know is that our friend has discovered that she is diabetic and, following her doctor's direction, began walking every day. She had to start gradually and work up. She now walks two miles every day and, in addition to helping her control her diabetes, her walk has become a high point of her day. She will readily tell you how beneficial exercise is and how much it has helped her not just physically but mentally.

Our purpose here is not to convince you that you should endure the physical pain of exercise to reap the gain. It is to encourage you to establish an exercise program in order to relieve the pain you may already be experiencing. The whole purpose of this book is to provide options for increasing pleasure, not pain, in sobriety. We are not going to discuss the benefits of exercise on your heart or lungs or for weight loss. You probably already know how important exercise is for your general health. Our purpose is to remind you of the benefits in reducing your stress by changing your brain chemistry. Certainly, exercise is important to your physical health. What we want to offer you is the pleasure reward that you can get from physical movement.

The truth is that physical activity can be fun, stimulating, and relaxing. A good exercise plan can add pleasure instead of pain to your life. The trick is finding a physical activity that is right for you, something you enjoy doing. No one sticks to an exercise program that is not enjoyable.

The more we move, the better we feel, the more motivated we are to move, and the more energy we have. We feel enlivened when we move. Movement allows us to feel our muscles work, our heart beat, and the blood flow through our bodies, creating energy and a feeling of well-being.

To Be Alive Is to Be Moving

"The unmoving water becomes the stagnant pool. The moving body freely channels the energy of life. Moving encourages movement. The more you move, the better you move. Energy creates energy—in a continuous, circling process—in a constant dance. Exercise makes us feel good—not just physically, but emotionally and spiritually. As if the physical advantages of exercise were not enough, its connection to the ways we think and feel about ourselves is remarkable. The moving body is the body releasing stress, letting go of pent-up emotions and unblocking channels for energy."

From *The Wellness Workbook*[3]

Many recovering people have found exercise to be extremely helpful in freeing them from the limitations of chronic abstinence symptoms. We know many recovering addicts who stop in the middle of their day's activities to exercise when they are feeling anxious or having difficulty concentrating or remembering. After exercising they feel much better and are more productive (and easier to get along with). Researchers at the University of North Carolina—Greensboro found that aerobic exercise reduces depression and anxiety levels in alcoholics.

Research indicates that exercise actually neutralizes brain chemicals that otherwise would increase craving for mood-altering substances. According to the National Center for Health Statistics, frequent exercisers have higher levels of endorphins and demonstrate more positive moods and less anxiety than those who exercise too little or not at all.

David: *Different forms of exercise have different payoffs for me. I have chosen these forms of exercise as strengthening contributions to my sobriety. Hiking or taking a long vigorous walk gives me special time to be completely alone with myself and my God, to meditate and to pray.*

I find that movement of my body up hills and down inclines in the heart of nature allows me to think more clearly, often resolving issues or making short-range plans. I find that a walk enables me to break out of the dull stupor that daily routine can bring. Because I automatically feel good while walking, my awareness of my surroundings is also sharpened as if a newly discovered sense is emerging. I then begin to think in a more positive way about myself and my life. I feel more in control of my life. By the end of the walk I am ready to meet new challenges with a new sense of inner strength.

Tennis relaxes me in another way. It provides strenuous exercise with almost every muscle being used with complete awareness of my physical self. It feels good to reach out and slam the ball, providing a surge of power and energy and anger release. Fellowship with my partner is also healthy and relaxing for me. Even though we are competing, it is all in fun. There is laughing, yelling, and just plain letting go.

Swimming is my special activity. I know of no other recreation that allows me more feelings of surrender. When I let go and become part of the water, I seem to flow through it with my worries and tension dissolving. Exercise is a vital part of my sobriety program and improves the quality of my life.

Aerobic Exercise

Regular exercise in which we use the whole body and keep moving at a steady pace—dancing, jogging, walking, swimming, bicycling—is aerobic and not only relieves stress and gives us a lift, but burns fat. Aerobic exercise increases oxygen intake. Increasing oxygen increases endorphins. While we do not recommend that you limit yourself to aerobic exercise, we strongly recommend that you participate in some aerobic activity every day. It is a good idea to have a variety of activities from which to choose so that an exercise plan is not dependent on partners or on the weather.

Walking is an excellent form of aerobic exercise that is usually readily available.. Walking can reduce tension and anxiety immediately. It is one of the most efficient forms of exercise and can be done safely throughout your life. It is also inexpensive and does not require special equipment other than good shoes. It offers the extra benefit of giving you time to reflect and organize your thoughts.

Walking can easily be incorporated into your daily activity. Maybe you can walk to work or to the bank, post office, or to visit a friend. Try taking the stairs instead of an elevator. Walk around the airport while waiting for your plane.

Stretching

Stretching exercises for warming up and cooling down will make your body more flexible. We recommend that you use stretching exercises throughout your day to relax muscles, reduce stiffness, and ease tension.

It is especially helpful to relax the muscles of your neck and shoulders throughout the day. Many people store a lot of tension in this area. Raise both of your shoulders at the same time and slowly rotate them in a circle, backward and then forward. Then roll your head around several times in a full circle as you keep your back straight.

Merlene Miller, MA and David Miller, PhD

Another place that many people store tension is in the lower back. To strengthen and relax those muscles, lie on your back with knees bent and feet flat on the floor. Tighten your abdominal muscles, grip your buttocks together, and flatten your lower back against the floor. Repeat this several times. Then bring one leg toward your chest. Pull the leg to your chest with your hands. Slowly curl your head toward your bent knee and hold for a count of five. Repeat the exercise with the other leg. Then do the exercise with both legs simultaneously. If you do these exercises for a few minutes every day, you will prevent or reduce much strain in your lower back.

Stress-Relief Tip

For a short tension reliever and also to improve circulation to the extremities, including the head, try placing the palms of your hands on your eyes for a few minutes. Follow this by placing your hands on the back of your head and twisting your body right and left while still seated. While your hands are still placed on the back of your head, touch each elbow to the knee on the same side and then back into the resting position.

Now, place one hand up and over behind your head, touching your back, and place the other hand on the opposite elbow and stretch. Alternately, bend the knees to the chest, one at a time, while sitting on a chair. Next, stretch by placing your feet and hands as far back on each side of the chair as you are able. Complete this exercise with a moment of relaxation by again placing your palms on your eyes and breathing deeply.

Diana W. Guthrie[3]

160

Fun, Laughter, and Play

Fun is a necessary part of life and of recovery, and it is often neglected. It is not only a part of recovery; it is an essential ingredient of life. Learning to enjoy life naturally will take time and practice because in the past fun has occurred unnaturally through mind-altering chemicals. So it will take some time to convince yourself that you do have the ability to have fun, to enjoy and celebrate without altering your mood artificially. You have the ability to create pleasure in natural ways. Fun and laughter relate directly to the production of endorphins. Fun is first and foremost a change of attitude, reaction, and perception about yourself as you slow down and experience life in the present.

Play is usually perceived as something separate and apart from life. Fun is seen as the icing of life; as long as you get your work done you can then, and only then, have fun. Life should be fun and fun a priority, not something we do when and if we have time. We can become so serious about staying sober that we never allow ourselves to have fun. Life without fun is like a long dental appointment. From time to time take breaks in your schedule that add color, spontaneity, and some zaniness to life. Put on your favorite music, sing, dance around the room, and let the child in you out. Have a water fight. Make yourself up like a clown. Get silly with the one you love. See what you can think of that is a little crazy and a lot of fun. Find people that you can have fun with; people that can let go and try new things.

Do you ever watch children having fun? They do not make a distinction between work and play. Play is their work. They play when they walk, talk, or when they are putting together puzzles. They are constantly using their developing senses to explore this new world and, for the most part are happy with their exploration. Don't let society's messages to act your age or grow up or stop being foolish deprive you of the richness of life that play offers. You may be so programmed to believe that playing is wasting time or that you need permission to play. Well, we give you permission. You must play for your health, your well being, and your recovery. You will find that you are able to accomplish more if you take time for play than if you neglect it.

Fun is its own reward. Fun feels good, and it enables us to feel good about ourselves. True enjoyment is characterized by laughter. Laughter releases feel-good brain chemicals and lightens our hearts. After we laugh we feel better, we think better, and we function better. Humor helps us adapt to change. Recovery requires a lot of change. Why not make it easier on yourself by seeing the humor and learning to laugh at yourself? Laughing at yourself allows you to give yourself permission to be imperfect. And when you can find humor in your own imperfections, it is easier to accept imperfections in others.

Research shows that laughter increases creativity and increases the ability to mentally organize information. Studies also show that humor, laughter, or mild elation enables people to remember, make decisions, and figure things out better. It seems this feel-good stuff is just what a person with chronic abstinence symptoms needs. Lighten up. Laugh a lot. It can only do you good.

Laughter is life's shock absorber. It allows you to take yourself lightly while taking other things seriously. Laughter is internal jogging, and you don't have to get dressed to do it. Look for things all around you to laugh about.

We can learn about play from children. Observe how they give themselves to each moment, allowing them to enjoy and experience whatever they are doing. We keep a notebook of funny things children in our family have said. Here are some favorites:

At Play
by David

Come, child, blend with me.
The time is now, as only time can be.
Come, child, let me share your world where pain is a stranger,
and glances laced with sweet innocence,
dance on a world made just for you.

Come, child, let me into your eyes.
Share your world where time has no back or front,
just a middle where all is now
as you contemplate some beauty of nature
cast in this plant or that bug.
Come, child, I will honor this time
where we may touch this now together,
as I learn of your wisdom
that I passed so blindly by on the path to "adult."

Come, child, allow me into your joyful laughter—
that clean innocent music where love and joy were born.
Come, child, remind me through your dancing eyes
of when I, too, was eternal and praised the world
through uncluttered observations, never mindful or
caring of expectations the world was casting my way,
dulling my senses through its call to sameness,
where wrong is to be different, where it's wrong to be me.

Come, child, teach me your ways once again
and allow me into your space to rest,
to find forgotten fragments of my self,
to reacquaint myself with the magic moment,
to be all that I can be—here and now.

- My teeth are shivering.
- God made me an eating person.
- You plug it in, and I'll plug it out.
- Why are you sleeping with your breakfast? (To someone eating in bed)
- I need a couple of water.
- A ghost is hollow on the inside and doesn't have any shell on the outside.
- Don't call Mom the old lady. She's no lady.
- Sometimes I snore when I laugh.
- Trix are for folks, too. You can have some; you're a folk.

Consider this old Japanese proverb, "Time spent laughing is time spent with the gods." Garrison Keillor says it this way. "Humor is not a trick. Humor is a presence in the world . . . like grace . . . and shines on everybody."

Pets

It is well-documented that pets can improve our health. Studies have shown that our enjoyment of our pets raises our spirits, lowers our blood pressure and cholesterol, and overall just makes life more enjoyable. Their unique, unconditional relationship with us helps us feel appreciated and important.

Did Someone Mention Pets?

Merlene: *Well, since you ask, we just happen to have pictures. Mazi is our amazing eight--pound papillion. In the last version of this book we told you about Sammy, our papillon who thought he was a great dane. We don't have Sammy anymore. We have Mazi who thinks she is a princess. And we do little to dissuade* her of that notion. She rules the house. She is a lap dog, and when she wants to be held she expects me to sit down and give her a lap. She wants to be with us all the time. But she quite often expects us to come where she is instead of coming where we are. She demands with a funny little sound that sounds like a cat. But we know that sound means she expects us to do her bidding. She doesn't like to drink out of a bowl because her ears get in the water, so she expects us to hold a glass of water for her while she drinks And like a small child she won't go to sleep at night without her drink. We keep her glass of water on the night stand. She also brings her rawhide stick to us to hold while she chews on it. People say she is spoiled. But David says, "What do I have to do that is more important than spoiling my dog?" One friend says that in his next life he wants to come back as our dog. She might be spoiled and she might be little, but Mazi is really big on heart. It's hard to believe so much love and affection can reside in so small a creature. She knows when we are sad or lonely or ill and she comforts us. We get a lot of return for spoiling her. Although she will only allow the two of us to pick her up, she loves everyone. She thinks that everyone who comes to the door comes to see her. She gets so excited she gets the zoomies, zipping around and around the house like she is propelled by a motor. Even the UPS man knows her by name and laughs at her antics. She runs to the door when we say, "Here comes Kevin." Of course she sleeps with us and curls up next to David like she is fastened with velcro. And when she wakes up in the morning the little princess rolls over for her belly rub. Since she has come into our lives, sleep has been more restful, laughter more frequent, and every day brighter. Although people say we are a little overzealous and spoil her a bit too much, most people who meet her admit that Mazi lights up the place. If you want to laugh more, love *more, be loved more, smile more, relax more, sleep better, or be happier, get a pet.*

Softening the Environment

Overload, high distractibility, hyper-vigilance, and stimulus augmentation all mean principally the same thing. When a person's filtering system does not work well, perception is altered. But you can learn to soften your environment and separate yourself periodically from unpleasant noises and sensations.

> **David:** *I may leave home without my American Express card. But I will never leave home without my earplugs! One of the best gifts of my life was a pair of earplugs given to me by a friend that works for General Motors. They have ridges on them that fit comfortably and snugly into the ear and, best of all, they work great. I can still hear with them in, but they soften the noise quite a bit so at least my nervous system doesn't spasm when that no-muffler car roars by.*

In addition to earplugs, a white-noise machine might be helpful. These ocean, or similar sound that covers up those clanging, banging noises. A fan or a computer may work because they both emit white noise of their own. Some people leave on the fan to their central air or furnace to give them constant white noise. Many of us are truly fans of fans.

You can also do things to quiet the environment where you live or spend time. Double-paned glass doors or windows and carpeting on the floor—or even on the wall—can deaden sound and allow some protection from unwanted sound intrusions. Learn to lower the noise levels in your environment. Tone down the music and turn off the television once in a while. The environment can also be softened with music; overstuffed furniture; simple, pleasant-to-the-eye décor; and harmonious colors.

> **Anne:** *I used to watch television to help me shut off my brain. But when I watched the news or a TV program, it seemed to disquiet my mind, and I would go to sleep more agitated. When I moved to Hawaii, I didn't take my TV with me. What I've learned is that TV did not shut off my brain—it gave me more things to think about.*
>
> *My apartment now is very quiet. Not having TV noise on makes a big difference. I feel more calm and relaxed without TV in my life. It has made all the difference in the world. It's as if the quietness has helped me to find an off button. I'm really at peace here. I feel centered, and I like that.*

You can learn to separate yourself periodically from the crowded stimuli you live with. Try putting a DO NOT DISTURB sign on the door. You can make time for quiet activities like browsing the libraries or museums. Or seek the quiet places in the great outdoors. In these ways you can temporarily eliminate noisy, chaotic activities.

> **Gale:** *Something that has often helped me is to go to a hot tub or a swimming pool where I float on my back. With my ears just under the water, I hear a roaring sound. The act of floating this way and the white noise that the water creates in my head relaxes and calms me and slows down my thought processes.*

But there are good sounds going on in the world, right along with the obnoxious ones. Most of the time, sounds of children playing and laughing can be pleasant. These playful sounds of life can be some of the greatest sounds of all, the sounds of living.

The perception of touch is also affected by stimulus augmentation. Letting people know to what extent you are comfortable being touched is important. It is also important to be comfortable physically with the right shoes and clothes.

> **Robin:** *Something that has helped me a lot with my stimulus augmentation is wearing comfortable clothing. When I have on tight or poor-fitting clothes, my stress levels go way up. It's not something most people think of when we talk about changing our environment. But it does make a difference.*

Touching

Touching in not just pleasurable; it is a human need. As we have tended to become isolated as a society—distanced as families and neighbors, whether because of the increased use of technology, the impersonal workplace, or our fear of crime and abuse—physical contact has suffered. The skin needs nurturing.

Skin is the body's largest organ and often the most neglected. Be good to your skin by wearing soft clothing made of natural fabrics that breathe. Protect it from sun damage. Use moisturizers to protect it from dryness. Touching is a great source of pleasure. Blood pressure can be lowered by petting a furry animal (especially one like Mazi). A hug can be very therapeutic. "Healing touch" is not just a phrase; it is an experience.

Enjoying Water

There is a natural healing power to water. We use water for hydration, cleansing, nutrition, relaxation, and recreation. It stimulates, warms, cools, soothes, and fulfills the need for touch.

Showering does more than cleanse. Use it to experience the healing power of water. Try standing under a shower and enjoying the feel of the water on your skin. To awaken your senses and increase circulation, alternate warm and cool water. Try a shower massager or shower at night with only a night light and imagine that you are standing in a waterfall.

Like a shower, a bath can also be used for more than cleansing. In the bath, water can touch you all over, can embrace you. It can soothe and relax you through its buoyancy, warmth, and gentleness. A hot tub provides much the same luxurious pleasure. In addition, its whirlpool jets can relieve an aching, sore body as well as soothe and relax muscles.

Swimming is one of few activities by which we can get complete exercise and a sensuous experience at the same time. Lap swimming can be meditative as well. If you wear goggles and earplugs, the sound of water gurgling as you swim contributes to the relaxation. Because the water supports every part of the body, this form of exercise can seem effortless. The water supports as it caresses.

It is not necessary to know how to swim to enjoy a dip in a pool. You can do water exercise or just splash and have fun. The weightless feeling is very pleasurable when you can let go and just be. Enjoy the buoyancy of the water by submerging yourself and floating to the top. There is nothing quite as luxurious as surrendering to the water by floating on your back, arms to your sides, eyes closed, and the water supporting you. Relax and feel the water surround you.

Music

Some sounds soothe and some invigorate. The sounds of music, waterfalls, rustling leaves, ocean waves, or birds singing are usually pleasing and enjoyable. Other sounds are pleasing to some people and not to other people. Be selective and choose sounds that help you feel more comfortable. Careful choice of music or sound can enhance the pleasure of daily life. It can brighten spirits or calm them down, depending on the type of music played.

Music is powerful. Music that is paced at fifty beats per minute is calming and relaxing. It can also provide a quiet background for study. Music energizes the body through vibration. Singing or humming is stress relieving. Music sets the stage for the body to be in balance and thereby supports the healing process.

> **David:** *A memorable magic moment occurred for me as I was going through a car wash. A Kenny G CD was on, and as I glided through the suds, I was cleansed by the sounds of the music; just rub-adub-dubbing along through the car wash, that sax and I were one. All around the car, music angels were flitting on swooshing wings delivering their rhythmic embrace, fusing me and settling an always fragile equilibrium with soothing resonance and artful elegance. I felt cleaner than the car, my sparkle enhanced by music's medicine.*

Music, art, and nature can be especially enjoyable for people with stimulus augmentation. Individuals with the ability to see and hear so much at one time often have an appreciation of details that simply pass others by. When listening to music they hear and experience every instrument. When looking at a painting they are aware of nuances of color not perceived by those less aware. When walking by the ocean they are aware of the sand beneath their feet, the color of the sky, the sound of the seagull, andthe grace of the pelican. They notice the size and shape of the shells, the roar of the sea, the regularity of the waves, and the great expanse of the water. And so they have the capacity to experience ecstasy and awe in a way that is unknown to those who can experience only one thing at a time.

Thirteen

STRESS-REDUCING ATTITUDES

While searching for ways to change your physiology and biochemistry to increase your comfort in sobriety, don't forget that how you feel is also determined by your thoughts, feelings, perceptions, perspectives, and beliefs. You are not a victim of your physiology. You are not powerless over your thoughts, feelings, and attitudes. You can choose how you look at yourself, other people, and the world. In doing so, you can improve your ability to handle stress and the challenges of recovery.

Anxiety Can Be an Opportunity

Anxiety is not necessarily bad. It can call your attention to a need for change, or it can make you mindful of something you've been unaware of. A crisis can be an opportunity.

The question is: Are you going to listen to what the anxiety is telling you or run from it? For many of us, anxiety triggers a desire to consume a substance that relieves anxiety. When this has been our way of reducing anxiety and we choose not to use that method anymore, we need other ways to decrease anxiety. If we don't find them, our level of anxiety continues to escalate.

You may believe that discomfort is proof that you are doing something wrong. Discomfort does not always mean that there is a problem. It may mean that something wonderful is about to happen. But to get to the other side of anxiety it is necessary to experience it and not try to make it go away. If you face it, it can help you discover what you believe about your situation, yourself, and your life. Pain can motivate you to move toward your dreams. But if your goal is to make it go away, you can usually find a way to do that—temporarily. If you can handle the discomfort without looking for pain control, then you may find yourself looking at a new opportunity.

Don't let anxiety get you off the track from where you want to go, whether your goal is staying sober or changing your career. Don't let fear block your dreams. The faith and courage you need to follow your dreams comes from the inner wisdom that knows what you need to do. When you listen to the voice that encourages you to go ahead, one step at a time, the anxiety lessens, and you can walk into opportunities you thought would always remain just dreams. Change demands risk, but change is an exciting part of life. Taking the risk to try something new keeps life exciting and full of surprises.

Sometimes anxiety is due to what we perceive is going on, rather than what is actually going on. We interpret events according to our perceptions. If we expect to be rejected, we may perceive that we have been, when in fact we haven't. If we believe ourselves incapable of doing a good job, we may think we are doing a poor job, when in fact we are doing well.

But anxiety does not always mean that something is wrong with your thinking; sometimes it means something is wrong with someone else's thinking. You can experience anxiety because others do not recognize or support your worth. In such situations, you might choose to avoid a crisis by accepting the other person's belief, but you experience anxiety when you settle for less than you deserve or are capable of.

There is a difference between feeling bad and being bad; the difference between fact and feelings. It is important to identify what your feelings are, respect them, and learn to express them in appropriate ways; but it is also important to recognize that these feelings may be based on inaccuracies. Sometimes, instead of changing our situation, we need to change our perception of it. In order to do that, it is necessary to tolerate discomfort long enough to figure out what the facts really are and what action is appropriate.

Learning to look at a situation differently can increase serenity even when there is nothing you can do to change it. Step back and refocus. Evaluate whether something is worth fighting for or about. Not every argument is worth trying to win. Set yourself free from the anxiety of unrealistic expectations.

Believe You Can Change

When we are unaware of effective ways to bring about change, we often apply the same would-be cures over and over again more intensely, more diligently. The more ineffective our actions, the harder we try, despite growing despair. If you are trying to pound a nail with a marshmallow, it doesn't help to hit harder. As you come to believe that nothing can be solved, you lose hope of anything getting better. A common statement that shuts out the possibility of change is "That's just the way I am." This is a way of saying, "Don't expect anything different from me. I will always be like I am."

Believing you can achieve something empowers you. This is not just the power of positive thinking. If you believe something is possible, you will invest more energy in making it happen than if you really don't believe it can happen. You have more energy to invest. Hope is energizing. It re-inspires confidence; it fires imagination and creativity. You do have choices, even when you don't know what they are. Feeling powerless is not the same as being powerless.

There are some payoffs in being powerless to change. Some of us get nurturing from being helpless; most of us do to some extent. Painful situations allow us to nurture ourselves in certain ways because we deserve it. After all, look at what we have suffered. We may believe we would have to give up nurturing ourselves if it was no longer a reward for our suffering.

Are people with an addiction victims? Well, in a sense, yes: victims of physiology. You didn't choose your body. If you were born that way, it certainly isn't your fault, and even those things you've done to contribute to the problem you did in the sincere attempt to make things better. People with addictions are also victims of public opinion and prejudice, but because this condition is not your fault does not mean you are not responsible for the choices you make as a result. It may be that heredity, your environment, and society have contributed to your situation. But, regardless of the contributing factors, you are the one that has to do something about it.

You can change. People change all the time. Change is a part of life. Believing you can do something not only gives you hope, it increases your chances for success. If you go to the gym and work out, you are not creating new muscles; you are just making the ones you already have stronger. The same is true for the abilities you need to change. You already have them. You just need to strengthen them. The most essential ingredient in the ability to change is courage. Courage is not lack of fear. It is taking action despite fear. It is being willing to risk failure or exposure. Many people are so immobilized by fear of failure that they live timid, cautious lives. They cannot act because they are so afraid of what will happen if they fail. If you want to develop courage, give yourself permission to fail. Courage gives you the freedom to try.

Accept Your Limitations

But believing you can change is not a magic answer. There are some things you can't change. You probably can't change the way your body responds to mood-altering substances when you ingest them. You probably can't change the way you metabolize alcohol when you drink. You can't change yourself into a 6'5" person if you are at your adult height of 5'4". There are some things that just *are*. When you can't accept some things as they are, you are always going to be frustrated. You will expend energy on things you have no power over, neglecting things you do have the power to change.

Anxiety can occur when you do not accept your limitations, when you fail to acknowledge that there are some problems you can't solve. The limitations that reality puts on us can be stressful. We cannot always be perfect. We cannot always be the best.

Mistakes are not failure. They're just mistakes. A mistake is not failure unless you refuse to learn from it. If you look at a mistake as an opportunity to learn rather than as failure, it can just be a step in your success. Most of us learn as much from what we do wrong as from what we do right. We learn what works and what doesn't work. We learn what to do differently the next time. Seeing mistakes as steps in the learning process allows us to use them as assets.

Applying the Serenity Prayer

Wisdom for recovery lies in the words of the Serenity Prayer: *God grant me the serenity to accept the things I cannot change, courage to change things I can, and wisdom* to know the difference.

Merlene Miller, MA and David Miller, PhD

Before you develop the serenity of acceptance or the courage to change, it is necessary to learn to tell the difference.

Learning about addiction and recovery will help you make responsible choices in relation to your condition. Numerous mistaken beliefs about addiction can lead to trying to change what you are powerless over. When you learn that chronic abstinence symptoms can be reduced by reducing stress, you can take action to change some stressful situations in life. The more you learn about addiction the better able you will be to make responsible choices.

With the process of recovery, there is the growing realization that the freedom to choose comes with continued sobriety. You are free to change your own behavior; mind-altering chemicals are no longer making your choices. With the freedom to choose comes responsibility. You are free to make responsible choices.

We create our own serenity by our attitudes and our spiritual resources. Serenity is a choice. You can fret about what you do not have the power to change—your heredity, the weathr, what is in the past, what isn't here yet, other people. Or you can accept those things and reinvest that energy in what you do have the power to control. Serenity is accepting what is and setting yourself free—joyfully—to experience the gift of life and the pleasures of sobriety.

Serenity does not mean you don't have any unpleasant feelings. It means you accept life as it is and do not expend excessive energy fighting against what you are powerless over. It does not mean that you do not get angry or afraid. Serenity means accepting and acknowledging all of your feelings. It is knowing that if you get angry you can handle it without hurting yourself or others. You can be serene and still be sad when your dog dies. Serenity is acceptance that your feelings are valid so you don't have to be ashamed or feel guilty about them.

Serenity is also knowing that what you feel and what you do about your feelings are not the same thing. You can be afraid and not run from what you are afraid of. You can be angry and not become violent. You can be sad and not give up on life. You can learn ways to express your feelings that are appropriate and healing.

Perhaps the real secret of serenity is in living in the present—being present in the moment. There is little serenity in replaying what has already happened or waiting for some time in the future to enjoy life. If you are living for tomorrow you are missing out on today. Serenity increases as the experience of being present and comfortable in the moment increases.

One day at a time is a slogan learned in AA that is helpful in recovery because it teaches one to focus on the present. Sometimes it can be broken down to one moment at a time. Now is all you have. The past is gone. You cannot change it. The future is not here yet. You cannot experience it. The present is where life is lived. Trying to live in the past or future robs you of the only life you have—the present.

Fourteen

ENRICHING LIFE

We all have a need for harmony in our lives; balancing our lives is living so that all parts are in harmony. While struggling with addiction your life may have become chaotic and unpredictable. At times you may have felt the insecurity of living on the edge—the edge of despair, the edge of giving up, the edge of complete loss of control. You may have felt the impact physically, mentally, emotionally, socially, and spiritually. You may have been out of harmony with yourself, others, and the world.

When we are focused on drinking or not drinking, we are out of balance, trying to do the impossible. Like a top that can't spin when it is not evenly weighted, we are drained of energy by our efforts to keep an unbalanced life in motion. When we are not getting as much energy from life as it drains from us, we are out of balance.

Balance creates energy; as we grow in recovery, we revitalize and rebalance all areas of our lives. We are released from attempting to achieve unattainable goals. Sickness and disharmony are replaced with wholeness and balance. We are revtalized, reconnected with healthy living. When we are living a balanced life, we are living responsibly, with time for family, job, friends, and ourselves. Balanced living includes attention to health care with proper focus on nutrition, exercise, and rest; to personal growth with proper regard to attitudes, feelings, and actions; to a healthy social network; and enriching spiritual life.

At first, recovery may seem chaotic. So much focus and attention on self-care may seem to put your life even more out of balance. It may seem that you are adding to an already-too-full schedule of activities, causing you to neglect other things that are important. But you cannot integrate good self-care into a balanced life until you learn the basic how-to's. Unavoidably, even in a life that is well balanced, special needs will arise and will cause you to focus on one aspect of living to the temporary exclusion of others. Beginning recovery is such a time. Learning good self-care habits and putting them into practice take time and energy, it's true, but after a while these practices become a predictable part of life.

As recovery becomes normal, you can move beyond basic self-care requirements—eating routines, exercise plans, and meetings. You can expand recovery. You will come to know yourself better while you become aware of the balance between too much and too little, responsibility to yourself and to others, time for work and time for play, time for activity and time for rest.

Balance of Body, Mind, and Spirit

We cannot look to any one aspect of life for all the answers. Because we are composed of many parts, we derive strength from many sources. Balanced living means we are healthy physically and psychologically and have healthy relationships. We recognize that each part of our lives impacts the others. We are no longer focused on only one aspect of life. We strive for and are motivated toward wholesome living.

Physical health allows psychological growth: When we feel good, we find it is easier to think about our attitudes and values and to work on eliminating shame, guilt, and anger. Psychological health allows us to do more easily those things that keep our bodies well. Healthy relationships support our personal growth.

But the whole is more than the sum of the parts. There is something more that is part of a whole person. Let's call it spirit. The spirit is more than just another part. It includes body, mind, feelings, behavior, and relationships, and it joins them all into a whole. The parts cannot be healthy until the whole is.

Balance Between Work and Play

Life is learning, and we learn better when we are having fun. For too many of us, fun is what we do when all the serious stuff (work) is done. Thinking this way keeps us imprisoned in the belief that we can live only on the weekends, on vacation, in retirement, or when we win the lottery.

Children do not make a distinction between work and play, they just experience life. Most adults have lost that ability. To the extent that we can recapture it, we allow ourselves to enjoy whatever we are doing, whatever we call it. Of course, we can't eliminate all activities that we do not especially enjoy; some tasks will resist being transformed from travail into treat. That is part of life. But it is still possible to enjoy a sense of accomplishment for doing them and to appreciate what we learn from the experience—and equally important, to give ourselves opportunity for the activities we do enjoy.

Merlene Miller, MA and David Miller, PhD

Balance Between Relaxation and Stimulation

Sometimes an unbalanced life means we need to learn to take life easier; sometimes it means we need more activities that stimulate and invigorate us. Rest is not doing nothing; it is enjoying the freedom to do anything.

We can be reenergized through both activity and inactivity. Some people prefer activities that excite; some prefer activities that relax.. Both types of activity do promote feelings of well being. But while all of us have our preference, most of us need some mixture of both types in order to live harmoniously with ourselves.

In recovery we may need to find new ways to feel calm or stimulated. Watching television or reading are good calming activities, but relaxation usually needs to be balanced by some activities that are physically stimulating (such as dancing) or mentally stimulating (playing a game or engaging in meaningful conversation). Relaxing means more than putting our feet up, although it certainly includes giving ourselves permission to do that. It also means getting our feet moving.

The balance of inactivity and activity also produces a balance of certain types of brain waves. When we are active, especially mentally active, we usually produce beta brain waves. When we are more mentally relaxed, we experience alpha and theta waves. Deep concentration produces a beta state; relaxation exercises produce an alpha or theta state. All mental states are essential to our total well-being, spending an inordinate amount of time in any one creates an imbalance. We create balance with variety in our activities.

Balance Between Giving and Receiving

For many of us, the most difficult aspect of our lives to balance is fulfilling our responsibility to ourselves and our responsibility to others.

Placing care of ourselves high on our list of priorities does not mean we do not also care for other people. Nor does giving to other people, even sacrificing for them, mean we should neglect our own recovery or our own growth. When we love ourselves, we take care of ourselves. When we love others, we allow them to take responsibility for their own lives as much as possible—but we support their growth, in whatever ways we can, without damaging ourselves.

As with other areas of recovery, our ability to provide for our own needs while responding to the needs of others expands as our recovery skills increase. At first, we may need to concentrate on our own needs as we learn to implement components of a self-care program. As those activities become a normal part of life, we are able to become more involved in supporting someone else. Paradoxically, giving often comes back to us as a gift.

Pass it on: *As her recovery expanded, Marilyn found that giving to others benefited her own growth. She put a sign in her car that read, "Pass It On," and often took people to the doctor, the grocery store, or AA meetings. She found time to listen when others needed someone to talk to. When anyone asked her what they could do to repay her, she said "Pass it on." Recently while a friend was in her home, Marilyn mentioned that she was unable to repaint her woodwork because she was allergic to the paint fumes. The friend said, "I'll paint your woodwork while you are on vacation and will air out your house before you get back." Marilyn was deeply touched that someone would offer to do that for her. The friend, seeing Marilyn's reaction, said, "I'm just passing it on."*

When we pass it on, we build a sense of community. When we just repay what has been done for us, we only balance the scales. The world is a better place to be when we are passing it on. A new energy is created that keeps on giving.

We need other people; our growth is dependent upon them. At the same time, we need to give to other people. We need to be concerned about others and contribute to their well-being. Through interaction with others we give and receive the feedback necessary for continuing growth. We cannot grow in a vacuum.

Many of us have not been able to achieve the balance of giving and receiving because we do not know how to love ourselves. Those of us who have lived in shame, who have felt defective and unacceptable, may feel unworthy of love and acceptance from others or from ourselves. When our recovery enables us to accept ourselves as we are, we are better able to have mutually supportive relationships with others.

We need strong social networks to nurture us and provide a sense of belonging. We need reciprocal relationships in which we feel valued as we value others and experience the satisfaction of giving and receiving.

Spiritual Balance

Spiritual balance means we are in harmony with ourselves, with our values, with others, and with God. Step Eleven of AA gives us guidance for achieving spiritual balance:

> *Sought through prayer and meditation to improve our conscious contact with God as we understood him, praying only for knowledge of His will for us and the power to carry that out.*

Just as we don't have to have any special concept of God to do this, neither do we have to use any certain definition of prayer or meditation. But this step is not about trying to get our higher power to do what we want. It is about aligning our will with a higher will. It is about getting in touch with a power that will help us increase our understanding, our knowledge, our courage, and our willingness to live wholesome lives.

Prayer does not change God, but
changes him who prays.

SØREN KIERKEGAARD

Spiritual wholeness is living in harmony with what we believe and value. Shame and guilt result from lack of harmony between our values and our behavior. Conscious contact with a higher power, increased knowledge of that power's will for us, and the power to carry that out enable us to find harmony between what we believe and what we do. We are thus freed from the burden of guilt and shame to find spiritual fulfillment.

Living in balance does not mean we do not have bad days. We still have our ups and downs; we still experience sadness, anger, fatigue, disappointment. We accept these feelings when they are appropriate. We don't have to be ashamed of them or feel guilty for having them. We allow ourselves to experience a whole range of feelings, but we don't let them control us. And we know how to take action that will prevent these emotions from triggering regression. A wholesome, harmonious life does not mean we never do things we regret or feel bad about. It means that we don't need to become discouraged by our inability to be perfect.

When we are living in balance, we accept our humanness and strive for progress. We seek to eliminate activities that cause us to go to extremes at the expense of other important parts of life. We give up the need for immediate gratification in order to achieve a lifestyle that is more fulfilling and meaningful. Harmony in all aspects of life allows us to go beyond the struggle of not using drugs and to enter into the experience of joyful living.

Joyful Living

Is there a voice within you, calling you to dream and to believe in your dreams? Listen to that voice. It is your creative spirit. It is calling you to live fully and passionately, to risk and to play. It is calling you to joy. As you listen to that voice and respond to it, it will become stronger. It is calling you to see yourself as a person of integrity and worth, one who has unique dreams and unique talents to offer the world. Responding to that special call leads us on a journey that goes beyond preventing relapse, beyond just getting back to ground zero. Seeing the possibilities of life and seeing ourselves with the potential for attaining wholeness gives purpose and meaning to our journey. That sense of purpose and meaning is a result and a facilitator of healing.

Replacing self-defeating lifestyles with hope and meaning takes self-care beyond maintenance into abundant living. Abundant living means more than material abundance. It means lives that are rich physically, mentally, socially, and spiritually. Moving beyond the issues of using or not using, we replace artificial ways of feeling good with natural ways. The brain creates positive chemistry and generates positive thoughts and feelings, leading to an expectation of opportunities and new possibilities. Life becomes an adventure.

We do not become aware of the possibilities for abundance if our main interest in life is the prevention of relapse. If we don't see something bright and new to move into, we can only long for what we are giving up. If we focus on an abundant life, and stay focused on it, then we will hope for that abundance, expect it, and seek it. If we feed our hopes, our fears will starve to death.

People who don't know how to live fully use temporary, artificial substitutes for the real riches life offers. But we know that in the long run these substitutes only increase pain, deadening senses rather than awakening them.

People who have used addictive living to produce pleasure or relieve pain and who don't know any other way to feel good or to relieve their pain, will eventually go back to addictive use. If our emphasis is on not drinking, then we're focused on what we are not doing; we're saying no to life. It is time we say yes—yes to living fully and joyfully.

A Spiritual Awakening

Step twelve of AA says: *Having had a spiritual awakening as a result of these steps, we tried to carry this message to others and to practice these principles in all our affairs.*

A spiritual awakening occurs as we go beyond the struggle of controlling our addiction and, having found meaning beyond ourselves, we discover the joys of living. We experience enriching pleasures that take us beyond just not using. We actively participate in life rather than passively hoping life will offer us something good along the way.

A spiritual awakening occurs as we learn that spirituality is not separate from our daily lives, but encompasses life and brings new meaning to all our affairs. Although spirituality must be defined by each of us for ourselves alone, it is interesting to note that Webster's dictionary tells us the word is derived from *spiritus*, which means "of breathing" and "an animating or vital principle held to give life." Our spiritual awakening allows this animating force to be breathed into all areas of our existence.

Spirituality and religion are not the same thing. Religion is a set of beliefs about the spiritual and the practices based on those beliefs. Religion certainly is a means by which some people connect to the spiritual, but we may experience a spiritual awakening without being affiliated with a specific religion. A spiritual awakening is a personal experience that opens the door to meaningful and creative living.

Living Creatively

When creativity is blocked, the result is powerlessness and impotence. To live creatively is to give expression to our inner selves. A creative spirit calls us to create laughter, love, forgiveness, and healing in ourselves and others. Creativity may be expressed through cooking, gardening, caring for children, caring for elderly, writing, playing, making love, decorating, painting, dancing, journaling, teaching, counseling, repairing, designing and so on.

The call to creativity is a call to joy, zest, and a sense of meaning and purpose. Are you listening to that call? Failure to experience life's meaningful pleasures creates a void that is often filled with destructive pleasures. They offer no hope and no joy.

We need to sharpen our senses rather than deaden them. We need to wake up and see what is already around us. Someone has said boredom comes from lack of involvement. Get involved. Celebrate life. Celebrate people and animals and all creation. Celebrate yourself.

We must learn to reawaken and keep ourselves
awake, not by mechanical aids, but by an
infinite expectation of the dawn, which does
not forsake us in our soundest sleep.

Henry David Thoreau

To live creatively and joyfully does not mean being happy all the time. Struggle is a normal and usually necessary part of creativity, just as labor is a normal part of giving birth. To live creatively is to experience a fullness of life; it is to be open to suffering as well as to pleasure. Pain is woven into life's pleasures and comforts, and is even essential to them. When we turn away from struggle, we turn away from progress, and a deeper pain grows. To escape from normal pain and struggle is to escape from life.

Compassion

Our pain can never be erased without compassion—"an awakening of passion with all creation."[1] Compassionate living means maintaining creative relationships with the earth, the creatures of the earth, and other people. The reason we damage the earth, one another, and ourselves is that we are out of harmony. Harmony results from valuing all creation, including ourselves—our bodies, minds, and spirits. Destructiveness comes from not honoring life. Compassion is reverence for life, including a reverence for our own specialness and our own beauty

> *The most beautiful experience we can have is the*
> *mysterious. It is the fundamental emotion which*
> *stands at the cradle of true art and true science.*
> *Whoever does not know it and can no longer*
> *wonder, no longer marvel, is as good as dead.*

ALBERT EINSTEIN

Compassion brings responsibility, not out of duty, but out of our wanting to care for what we cherish and value. What do you cherish? What are you enthusiastic about? The word *enthusiasm* means "spirit." Do you have life-spirit? Do you have self-spirit? Compassion is a call to courage. Discouragement kills faith and hope and spirit. Courage awakens and empowers. It empowers us to walk into our dreams with hope and enthusiasm.

An important aspect of recovery is giving to others out of compassion and concern. Our own wounds become a resource for healing: Out of our suffering come the wisdom and understanding to pass the healing on. Those of us for whom addiction has been the object and focus of life have the opportunity to give to others in recovery. Having lived through much anguish, we are survivors of a condition that has eaten the very center out of our self-esteem. Out of this struggle, we gain insight and compassion to give to and receive from others. Sharing these principles with others is important in keeping them active in our own lives.

Nothing renews commitment like sharing
the joy that results from the commitment . . .
sharing keeps the light on and the spirit high.

LARRENE HAGAMAN[2]

Sharing with others keeps the growth going. Without it we retreat back into oujr old selves and allow the old shames to creep in and take over. Carrying the message allows life to take on an "other" focus rather than just a "self" focus. As we give to others, we reflect their worth and see our own worth reflected in them. This sense of unity creates a deeper sense of the interconnectedness we have with others and with all living things

Freedom

Freedom of choice is the greatest opportunity we have. We can choose life; we can choose to take a different path no matter where we have been. We can choose to use the resources we have to become what we were created to be. Or we can choose to hang on to feelings of inadequacy that keep us locked into discouragement.

As we become aware of our ability to use our own judgment and, through that exercise, to assert more control over our own lives, we begin to see our potential instead of our shortcomings. We stop seeing other people through defensive eyes as we learn to see them in the light of our empowering interaction with them. We see that we, as individuals working and playing together, can become more than we could in isolation.

We really do not grow or gain in self-esteem by adhering to the wisdom of the self alone. We need, ultimately, to feel a sense of belonging. We need to be involved with others, to exchange perceptions with them, to give and get support. We need others to help us stop the inner war that is fueled by shame and distorted pictures of ourselves.

Freedom comes from an emphasis on what we are seeking rather than on what we are avoiding. If emphasis is on the not (what we are not consuming, what habits we are not engaging in), then we are always aware of what is lacking in our lives. Life seems to mean deprivation and restriction. But as we move into replacement activities we expect abundance. Armed as never before against regression, we are freed to spiral up into new aspects of growth.

Serendipity

A bonus on the recovery journey, serendipity is the good fortune of discovering something good while seeking something else. It happens when we compare what we have been seeking with what we have found, and decide that the thing we've found is even better than that which we'd sought. Many people, out of their pain and acceptance, have experiences in which their insights and benefits far surpass their expectations of merely staying on track.

The person at an AA meeting who says "I'm a grateful alcoholic" is describing this experience of serendipity. She has found on her healing journey much more than she ever expected, more than only maintaining abstinence, more than just hanging on. A new way of life has opened up for her. Expecting serendipity means living in a way that says, "Today I can experience only the present. As I do, I expect the unexpected. I have a choice to truly experience today, as fully as I can."

A certain story has held particular meaning for us, and we wish to share it with you. We hope it will help light the path that you take in recovery.

There was once a young farm boy whose father was away and whose mother asked him to go to the barn in the dark to feed the animals. But he was afraid of the dark. His mother assured him that the flashlight would furnish the light he needed to get there and back. "But the light only shines a short way in front of me," he said. "I can't see all the way to the barn." Then his mother took him outside. "Now, son," she said, "just take one step toward the barn." As he took one step the light moved ahead of him. "All you have to do," his mother told him, "is take one step at a time and the light will go before you all the way."

There is a light that goes ahead of us on our recovery journey. We can see as far as we need to see to live a full and joyful life. We don't have to wait until we get to the end of the journey to begin living or to experience the light. As you take your next steps into recovery, watch for the light that illuminates your path.

Appendix
A Scientific Trieste Leading to Dopamine Homeostasis

We review here the scientific history of the development of a dopamine optimization complex called KB220 to provide for the eventual balancing of the brain reward system and the induction of dopamine homeostasis.

In 1968 Blum and Geller received a grant from the National Institute on Alcohol Abuse and Alcoholism (NIAAA) to do animal research into the rolel of neurotransmitters in stress and aberrant alcohol drinking. They found that serotonin was involved in drug seeking behavior by evoking the concept of darkness-induced drinking based on the effect of pineal gland melatonin, a substance found in the brain synthesized from serotonin. From 1968-1972 the research focused on the role of stress-induced changes in brain chemistry.

During this time Blum and his associates provided data that supported the concept of shared neurochemical mechanisms between alcohol and opiates by showing that the narcotic antagonist naloxone blocked alcohol dependence in mice. This finding led to the clinical development of vivitrol (Naltrexone) used currently as an FDA approved pharmaceutical to treat both alcoholism as well as opiate addiction.

Dr. Blum's group was the first to identify a metabolite isoquinolones (a combination of the acid form of alcohol and dopamine) in the brain of mice following ethanol ingestion, which helped support the common mechanism theory of alcohol and opiates.

In the late 70's and early 80's Blum dedicated his research to endorphinergic research and was the first group to show the unequivocal role of methionine–enkephalin (METENK) as the basis for alcohol intake. Specifically, low METENK induced high ethanol drinking and vica versa high METENK induced low ethanol intake.

Concurrently the concept the genes might be one reason why some people cannot control was developed. The question was also asked whether the environment as well as genetics could be involved. In1982 Dr. Blum published his seminal work in *Science* showing that ethanol drinking in Golden Syrian hamsters freely drinking for one year (equivalent to 20 years in humans) had very significant impairment in striatal leucine-enkephalin synthesis. This finding has been confirmed in humans and shown by others to occur with chronic intake of opiates, diazepam and cocaine.

Other work revealed that intra-cerebellum injections of enkephlamide (a methyl analog of enkephalin) induced a significant reduction of ethanol intake in high ethanol seeking C57/blk mice.

Blum and his associates found that by inhibiting carboxyl- peptidase (basically enkephalinase) D-Phenylalanine for 18 days in C57/blk alocohol loving mice, endorphin levels were raised in both the pituitary and striatum and caused the genetically prone alcohol-seeking mice to significantly reduce their alcohol intake to similar levels of non-preferring alcohol mice.

This work, published in the journal *Alcohol* provided the starting point for the role of enkephalinase inhibition as a therapeutic target for the treatment of alcoholism.

In 1982 Blum then began to develop KB220, experimenting with a male human alcoholic realizing that an anti-alcoholic agent must constitute a number of select precursor neurotransmitter-based amino–acids; an enkephalinase inhibitor and inhibitors of both mitochondrial and synaptic enzymes which catabolize (breakdowown enzymes) catecholamines such as serotonin and dopamine.

Following many iterations the first ever neuronutrient was formulated and resulted in successful reduction of heavy drinking in a male alcoholic. Further reiterations also resulted in successful amelioration of serious drinking in a female alcoholic.

Over the next eight years the first commercialization of this neuronutrient KB220 (called SAAVE) was utilized in over 1,000 treatment centers in the USA. Blum's group continued to develop related formulations for cocaine dependence (Tropamine), opiate dependence (SAAVE PLUS) and even obesity (PhenCal).

During this period many research papers related to clinical outcomes including double–blind placebo investigations appeared in the scientific literature. The response from the recovery community was very positive and as such amino-acid therapy for the treatment of drug addiction was born.

Blum along with Gerald Kozlowski of Southwestern Medical School in Dallas began to track the various ways the neurotransmitters interact in the brain. This basic research resulted in the development of the understanding of the well-known reward circuitry of the brain whereby they coined and published in 1989 the term *"Brain Reward Cascade"* (BRC).

Many investigations by global scientists over the last 25 years have supported this basic conceptual framework, has stood the test of time, and is considered a blueprint of neurotransmitter interaction and subsequent workings of the reward system and reward dependent behaviors. The basic tenant of this work revealed that the feeling of well-being can be achieved only when the molecule dopamine is released in the nucleus accumbens at homeostatic levels. Any deviation causes *dopamine resistance* and as such could result in aberrant cravings. Specifically, too much dopamine can lead to schizophrenia and too little dopamine could lead to depression.

Following this research Blum's group turned their attention to unraveling the long known concept that alcoholism was an inheritable disorder but was lacking any specific studies. Along with Ernest

Merlene Miller, MA and David Miller, PhD

P. Noble, the former director of NIAAA and Pscychiatric Professsor at UCLA Blum began to analyze brain tissue from both alcoholics (80% cirrhosis of the liver) and non-alcoholics loking for genes that affect the Brain Reward Cascade. Restriction Fragment Length Polymorphism (RFLP) techniques to discover the first ever genetic association of alcoholism. They published their findings in JAMA in 1990, showing the now famous association of the dopamine-D2–receptor gene (DRD2) A1 allele (variant) with severe alcoholism.

Initially, this astounding discovery met with controversy worldwide but is now considered a major breakthrough in addiction medicine and has been researched in almost 4,000 scientific studies cited in PUBMED. In fact, the JAMA study sparked the entire field known as "Psychiatric Genetics."

Subsequent to their finding Noble, Blum and associates were the first to report that carriers of the DRD2 A1 allele were born with a 30-40% lower number of D2 receptors and as such are at high risk for all addictive behaviors both substance and non-substance related. Currently the DRD2 gene is considered to have significant on all reward behaviors and as such has been considered a "reward gene."

In 1995, understanding the nature of common neurogenetic and neurobiological mechanisms shared across the major abusable licit and illicit drugs and the importance of a hypodopaminergic trait/state, Blum first conceived and coined the term "Reward Deficiency Syndrome"(RDS) to describe addictive, impulsive disorders including alcoholism, drug abuse, attention deficit disorder, gaming, internet addiction, sex addiction, and food bingeing, having a common genetic basis acting as an umbrella term.

One important outcome derived from this work resulted in a paper by Blum's group published in the Royal Society of Medicine revealing that carriers of the DRD2 A1 allele variant have a 74.4% predictive risk for RDS.

In unpublished work, Blum and associates show significant predictability of a ten-gene reward panel to associate with ASI-Media Version alcohol and drug severity scores. This genetic test called Gentic Addiction Risk Score (GARS) can precdict genetic risk for the development of addiction.

Since the 80's until the present time Blum's group has published close to 30 peer-reviewed articles showing clinical benefits of NAAT. The major highlight of this work has been focused on the utilization of neuroimaging tools. In a series of articles it was shown that NAAT caused significant regulation in the pre-frontal cortices especially at the cingulate gyrus (a region for drug relapse) in abstinent psychostimulant abusers, alcoholics, and opiate addicts utilizing qEEG analysis following both intravenous and/or oral administration within one hour following administration of NAAT.

Most recently in a placebo controlled cross over study NAAT significantly restored resting state functional connectivity in abstinent heroin addicts across a putative network including the dorsal anterior cingulate, medial frontal gyrus, nucleus accumbens, posterior cingulate, occipital cortical areas, and cerebellum.

In other unpublished rat work it has been also shown that NAAT significantly activates, above placebo, seed regions of interest including the left nucleus accumbens, cingulate gyrus, anterior thalamic nuclei, hippocampus, pre-limbic and infra-limbic loci.

Blum's group has also now published in peer reviewed journals the complete elimination of terrifying PTSD-induced nightmares following administration of NAAT.

This summary of research and the development provides solid scientific support for the utilization of NAAT therapy.

For more information on some of the therapies mentioned in this book or additional copies of this book call: **800-614-7714**

Notes

Chapter 2

1. D. Smith, "The process of addiction and the new ASAM definition of addicrion, " *J Psychoactive Drugs,* (Jan-Mar 2012) 44(1):1-4

2. M. Gold, et al., "A Shared Moleculare and Genetic Basis for Food and Drug Addiction: Overcoming Hypodopaminergic Trait/State by Incorporating Dopamine Agonist Therpay in Psychiatry," *Psychiart Clin North Am,* 38(3):419-62.

3. M. Paulus, "Neural activation patterns of methamphetamine dependent subjects during decision making predict relapse, "Arch gen psychiatry, (2005), 62(7):761-8.

4. K.Blum, et al., "Neurogenetic and epigenetic correlates of adolescent predisposition to and risk for addictive behaviors as a function of the prefrontal cortex dysregulation, *J Child Adolesc Psychopharmacol,* (May 2015), 25(4):286-92.

5. K. Blum, et al., "Reward deficiency syndrome: a biogenic model for the diagnosis and treatment of impulsive, addictive, and compulsive behaviors, "K. Blum, et al., *Reward deficiency syndrome:a biogenic model for the diagnosis and treatment of impulsive, addictive, and compulsive behaviors." J Psychoactive Drugs,* (Nov 2000), 32 Suppl:i-iv, 1-112.

6. K. Blum, et al., "Generational association studies of dopaminergic genes in reward deficiency syndrome "RDS" subjects:selecting appropriate phenotypes for reward dependence behaviors, " *Int J Environ Res Public Health,*(Dec 2011) 8(12):4425-59.

7. K. Blum, et al., "The D2 dopamine receptor gene as a determinant of reward deficiency syndrome, *J R Soc Med,* (Jul 1996(89)7:396-400.

8. K. Blum, et al., "Neurogenics and gene therapy for reward deficiency syndrome: are we going to the promised land? " *Expert Opin Biol Ther,* 15(7):973-85.

9. K. Blum, "Allelic association of human dopamine d2 receptor gene in alcoholism, " *JAMA,* (Apr 1990) 18:263)15:2055-60.

10. E Nestler, et al., "Epigenetic basis of mental illness, " *Neuroscientist,* pii:1073858415608147.

11. H.Szutorisz, et al., "Parental THC exposure leads to compulsive heroin seeking and altered striatal synaptic plasticity in the subsequent generation," N*europsychopharmacology,* (May 2014), 39(6):1315-23.

12. K. Blum, "Reduced leucine-enkephalin-like immunoreactive substance in hamster basal ganglia after long-term ethanol exposure, " *Science,* (Jun 1982) 25;216(4553):1425-7.

13. K. Blum, "Hatching the behavioral addiction egg; Reward Deficiency Solution System (RDSS)™ as a function of dopaminergic neurogenetics and brain functional connectivity linking all addictions under a common rubric," *J Behav Addict, 149-56. doi:10.1556/JBA.3.2014019.*

14. A.Gyollai, "The genetics of problem and pathological gambling; a systematic review, " *Curr Pharm Des,*(2014) 20(25):3993-9.

Chapter 4

. National Drug Intelligence Center online National Center on Substance Abuse online. National Center on Addiction and Substance Abuse online. For more information about Alcoholics Anonymous, see: *Alcoholics Anonymous.* (Alcoholics Anonymous World Services, Inc., 1955). *Narcotics Anonymous.* (C.A.R.E.N.A. Publishing Co., 1982)

2. For more information about the disease model of alcoholism, see: Maltzman, "Why Alcoholism Is a Disease," *Journal of Psychoactive Drugs* 26 (1994): 13-31. James Milam, "The Alcoholism Revolution," *Professional Counselor* 8 (1992). Kenneth Blum and James Payne, *Alcohol and the Addictive Brain.* (New York: The Free Press, 1991).

3. For more information on these symptoms, see:

4. Terence Gorski and Merlene Miller, *Staying Sober: A Guide for Relapse Prevention.* (Independence, MO: Herald House Independence Press, 1986). Merlene Miller and David Miller. *Reversing the Regression Spiral,* (Miller Associates, 2012).

5. *Alcoholics Anonymous.* (Alcoholics Anonymous World Services, Inc., 1955).

6. Katherine Ketcham and William Asbury, *Beyond the Influence.* (New York: Bantam Books, 2000).

Chapter 5

1. K. Blum, et al., "Neurogenetics and nutrigenomics of nuro-nutrient therapy forr Reward Deficency Syndrome (RDS):

Clinical ramifications as a function of molecular neuurobiologicl mechanisms," *J Addict Res Ther* (Nov 2012): 27:3(5) 139.

2. K.Blum, et al., "Hypothesizing ealancing endorphinergic and glutaminergic systems to treat and prevent relapse to reward reficiency behaviors: boupling D-Phenylalamine and N-Acetytl-Cysteine (NAC) as a Therapeutic Modality," *Clin Med Rev Case Rep:* (2015): 2(8) pii o76.

3. TJ Chen, et al., "Neurogenics and clinical evidence for the putrative activation of the brain reward circuitry by a neuroadaptagen: Proposing addiction candidate gene panel map," *J Psychoactive Drugs* 43(2):108-127.

4. K. Blum, et al, "Enkephalinase inhibition tegulation of ethanol intake in genetically predisposed mice," *JE* (1987) 4(6):449-56.

5. T, Yamaguhi, et al., "Mesocotyiolimbic Ggutamatnergic pathway," *J Neurosci*, (2011) 31(23)::8476-90.K. Blum, et al., Manipulation of Cataecho-O-Methyl-Transferase (COMT) activity to influence the attenuation of substance seeking behavior, A subtype of Reward Deficiency Syndrome (RDS), is dependent upon gene polymorphisms: A hypothesis," *Med Hypothesis*, (2007) 69(5):1054-60.Y. Hua, et al., "Molecular mechanisms of chromium in alleviating insulin resistance," *J Nutr Biochem* (2012) 23(4):313-9

6. Joan Mathews-Larson, 7 *Weeks to Sobriety.* (New York: Fawcett Columbine, rev. ed., 1997) Charles Gant, *End Your Addiction NOW.* (New York: Warner Books, 2002).
J. Ross, *The Diet Cure.* . (New York: Penguin Group, 1999).
J. Ross, *The Mood Cure.* (New York: Penguin Group, 2002).

7. David Miller, et al, "Addiction Treatment in America: After Money or Aftercate?" *Reward Deficiency Syndrome,* (2015): 1(3):87-94.

8. Merlene Miller, et al, "Early Intervention of Intravenous KB200IV, Neuroadaptagen amino-acid therapy) NAAT improves behavioral outcomes in a Residential Addiciton Treatment Program: A Pilot study.," *J Psychoactive Drugs,* 44(5):384-40

9. Kenneth Blum, et al, "Genetic Evidence for Predisposition to Reward Deficiency Syndnrome (RDS)," *Mol Neurobiol,* (2014) 50(3)

Chapter 6
1. B.A. Watkins, et al., "Food lipids and bone health," in *Food Lipids and Health,* R.E. McDonald and D.B. Min, eds. (New York: Marcel Dekker, 1996), pp. 101-02.

2. G.H. Dahlen, eat al., *journal of Internal Medicine* 244(5) (Nov 1998): 417-24.

3. P. Khosla and K.C. Hayes, J*ournal of the American College of Nutrition* 15 (1966): 325-39.

4. B.A. Clevidence, et al., *Arteriosclerosis, Thrombosis, and Vascular Biology* 17 (1997): 1657-61,

5. M.L. Garg, et al., *Federation of American Societies for Experimental Biology Journal* 2 (4) (1988): A852.

6. L.D. Lawson and F. Kummerow, "Lipids," 14 (1979): 501-03.

7. M.L. Garg, *Lipids* 24(4) (April 1989): 334-39

8. Presented by Sarah M. Conklin, Ph.D., Cardiovascular Behavioral Medicine Program, University of Pittsburgh, at the American Psychosomatic Society's Annual Meeting, Budapest, Hungary, March 2007.

9. For more information on the health benefits of coconut oil, see: A. Keys, et al., "The diet and 15-year death rate in the seven countries study." *American journal of Epidemiology,*(1986) 124: 903-15.

10. LA. Prior, et al., "Cholesterol, coconuts, and diet on Polynesian Atolls: A natural experiment: the Pukapuka and Tokelau Island studies," *American Journal of Clinical Nutrition 34(8)* (1981): 1552-61.

11. Bruce Fife, *The Healing Miracles of Coconut Oil.* (Colorado Springs, CO: Health Wise, 2001), 20-23.

12. Weston Price, *Nutrition and Physical Degeneration* (Keats Publishing, 1998).

13. W. Willett, "Diet and coronary keart disease." *Monographs in Epidemiology and Biostatistics* (1990) 15: 341-79.

14. World Health Organization. "Diet, Nutrition, and the Prevention of Chronic Diseases. Report of a WHO Study Group." *WHO Technical Report Series* 797, Geneva, Switzerland, 1990.

Chapter 8

1. M.B. Sterman, "EEG biofeedback: physiological behavior modification," *Neuroscience and Biobehavioral Reviews* 5, No. 3 (1981): 405-12.

2. J. Lubar, et al., "Evaluation of the effectiveness of EEG neurofeedback training for ADHD in a clinical setting, as measured by changes in T.O.V.A. scores, bBehavioral ratings, and WISC-R performance," *Biofeedback and Self-Regulation* 21, (1995): 83-99.

3. M.B. Sterman and L. Friar, "Suppression of seizures in an epileptic following sensorimotor EEG feedback training," *Clinical Neurophysiology* 33 (1972): 89-95.

4. M.B. Sterman, et al., "Biofeedback training of the sensorimotor EEG rhythm in man: effect on epilepsy," *Epilepsia* 15 (1974): 395-416.

5. For more information about Beta Training Neurofeedback, see: V.J. Monastra, et al., "Assessing attention deficit hyperactivity disorder via quantitative electroencephalography: an initial validation study," *Neuropsychology* 13 (1999): 424-33.

6. M.A. Tansey, "Righting the rhythms of reason: EEG biofeedback training as a therapeutic modality in a clinical office setting," *Medical Psychotherapy* 3 (1990): 57-68.

7. *Colorado Springs Gazette,* April 29, 2004.

8. For more about the Alpha-Theta Protocol, see: E.G. Peniston and P.J. Kulkosky, "Alcoholic personality and alpha-theta brainwave training," *Medical Psychotherapy* 4 (1991): 1-14.

9. T. Stephenson, "Link between memory and neurofeedback," *Imperial College London Reporter* 126 (February 5, 2003).

10. Connie Higley and Alan Higley, *Reference Guide for Essential Oils.* (Olathe, KS: Abundant Health, 1998).

11. Isadore Rosenfeld, *Dr. Rosenfeld's Guide to Alternative Medicine.* (New York: Random House, 1996).

Chapter 11
1. Jack Trimpey, *The Small Book.* (New York: Dell Publishing, 1989).

Chapter 12
1. January 1996.

2. Regina Sara Ryan and John W. Travis, *The Wellness Workbook.* (Berkeley, CA: Ten Speed Press, 1981).

3. Diana W. Guthrie, *Alternative and Complementary Diabetes Care.* (New York: John Wiley and Sons, Inc., 2000).

Chapter 14
1. Matthew Fox, *The Coming of the Cosmic Christ.* (San Francisco Harper and Row, 1988): 32.

2. Larrene Hagaman, "Building the Temple Within," *The Restoration Witness* (September/October 1990): 4-12.